Contents

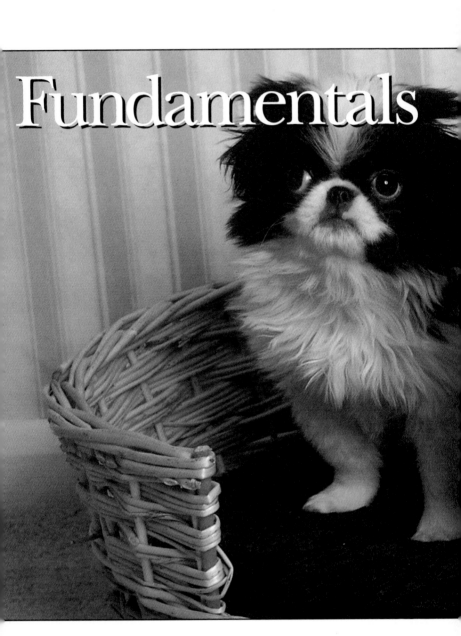

Fundamentals

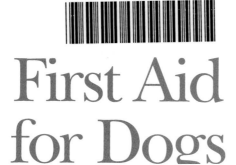
First Aid
for Dogs

Owner's Guide To

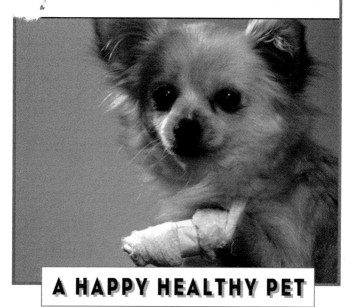

A HAPPY HEALTHY PET

Howell Book House

Howell Book House
A Simon & Schuster Macmillan Company
1633 Broadway
New York, NY 10019

Library of Congress Cataloging-in-Publication Data
Schwartz, Stefanie.
First aid for dogs/Stefanie Schwartz.
—An owner's guide to a happy healthy pet
  p. cm.
ISBN 0-87605-565-X

1. Dogs—Wounds and injuries—Treatment.   2. Dogs—Diseases—Treatment.
3. Veterinary emergencies.   4. First aid for animals.   I. Title.   II. Series.
SF991.S324   1998   98-16858
636.7'08960252—dc21   CIP

Series Director: Amanda Pisani
Assistant Series Director: Jennifer Liberts
Book Design: Michele Laseau
Cover Design: Iris Jeromnimon
Illustration: Casey Price
Photography:
  Front cover by Winter Churchill Photography
  Front cover inset by Paulette Braun (Pets by Paulette)
  Back cover by Daniel Wallace
  Joan Balzarini: 16, 96, 99
  Cheryl Primeau: 19, 38, 46, 67, 73, 86, 101
  Bob Schwartz: 2–3, 5, 6, 12, 15, 20, 35, 37, 44–45, 48, 54, 60, 68, 71, 77, 84, 88, 94, 102, 107, 114, 124
  Stefanie Schwartz: 89
  Judith Strom: 87, 93, 116
  Toni Tucker: 63
  Faith Uridel: 69
  Daniel Wallace: 10, 11, 17, 26, 30, 31, 32, 43, 49, 51, 52, 58, 65, 66, 74, 75, 85, 90, 92, 100, 109, 118, 119, 121, 122
  Jean Wentworth: 23
  Winter Churchill Photography: i
Production Team: Stephanie Mohler, Clint Lahnen, Angel Perez, Dennis Sheehan, Terri Sheehan

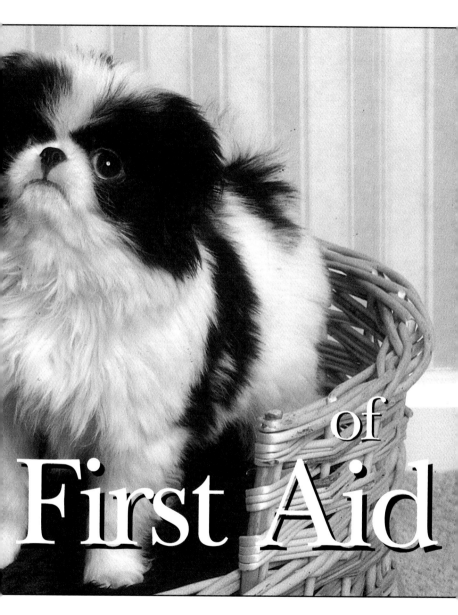

First Aid
of

Skeletal System of a Dog

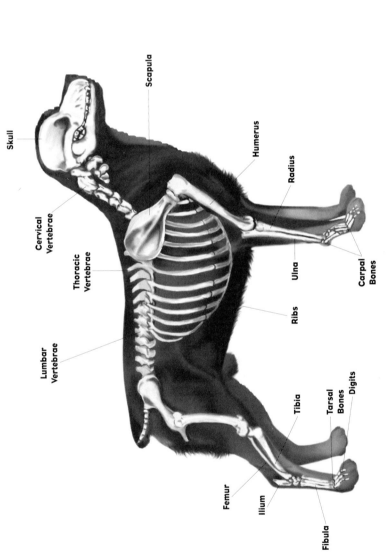

Skull

Cervical Vertebrae

Thoracic Vertebrae

Lumbar Vertebrae

Scapula

Humerus

Radius

Ulna

Carpal Bones

Ribs

Femur

Ilium

Tibia

Tarsal Bones

Digits

Fibula

chapter 1

What Is

First Aid?

"First aid" is the first response to aid a dog in an emergency situation. Depending on the specific injury or illness, the dog may need only simple intervention to become stabilized. At the other extreme, there may be little anyone can do at the scene and immediate transfer to the nearest veterinary facility may be the best first aid.

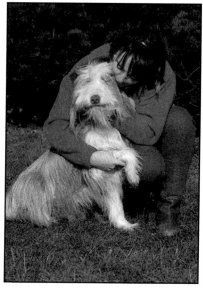

There are many types of emergencies and some are more immediately life-threatening than others. Compare, for example, the severity between a dog that has broken his tail with a dog that has been hit by a car. A tail is not a vital organ and although the injury may be quite painful, it is unlikely to be life-threatening. A dog that has been hit by a car can suffer injuries that may range from minimal (perhaps only a few scrapes) to severe (such as internal bleeding) if the dog is lucky enough to survive the impact at all.

The Goals of First Aid

The primary goal of first aid is to take immediate and appropriate action to preserve the life of the patient.

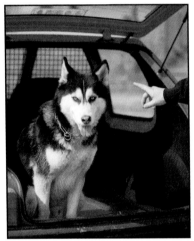

First aid is most valuable in extreme emergency situations when failure to respond could result in the dog's death.

The second goal of first aid is to prevent further deterioration of the dog. As soon as a physical problem becomes apparent, appropriate intervention is required to keep things from getting worse until trained professionals have an opportunity to intervene.

The third goal of first aid is to relieve pain and discomfort. Pain is

In almost every case, first aid should not replace veterinary attention. When in doubt, take your dog to the veterinarian for treatment.

not necessarily a reliable indication of the severity of an injury or illness. Causing some pain to an injured dog may be unavoidable during first aid, for example, when the dog is gently lifted into your car for transport to the clinic. Moreover, it might not be advisable to relieve pain completely in an injured animal as the dog will likely try to move around before healing is complete.

And finally, the fourth goal of first aid is to ensure the health of the dog with immediate veterinary attention. The purpose of this book is not to teach everything there is to know about veterinary emergency medicine and care. As a devoted and concerned dog owner, it is important that you understand the basics of the most commonly encountered veterinary emergencies. In many situations, you will be able to make a difference by responding appropriately to help your sick or injured pet. But unless you are a veterinarian, you should not make decisions regarding your pet's safety or survival without the benefit of first-hand veterinary attention. First aid should be directed at your dog's initial care in the actual emergency situation or as soon as a problem is discovered. In almost every case, first aid should not replace subsequent veterinary attention.

First Aid Kit

The following items are easily obtained from your local pharmacy. You should store them in a moistureproof container that is easily accessible in an emergency (but out of reach of children and pets). In addition, include a list of emergency telephone numbers on an index card. You may want to have this laminated or place it inside a plastic cover. You might also include a copy of this book for quick reference as necessary. Think about making a duplicate kit to keep with you in the car in case something happens when you are away from home. If you often travel with your dog, research the availability of emergency veterinary coverage at your destination. The better prepared you are, the less likely you are to panic in case of an emergency.

Practice Before an Emergency

Practicing before an emergency can be a vital investment:

- The more comfortable you are in using the contents of the first aid kit, the more smoothly you can respond should the need arise.

THE CONTENTS OF YOUR FIRST AID KIT

- 2 rolls of gauze: 1 that is 2 inches wide and 1 that is 3 or 4 inches wide
- 1 roll of white "surgical" tape, 1 inch wide
- 2 rolls of elastic wrap, 1 that is 2 inches wide and 1 that is 3 or 4 inches wide
- 1 roll of cotton batting (12 inches wide)
- an emergency ice pack
- a bottle of 1 percent hydrogen peroxide
- a box of latex examination gloves or alternative gloves
- an extra collar and leash
- a soft muzzle; alternatively, a smooth nylon rope (about 2 to 3 feet long) or an old pair of panty hose can be tied for use as a soft muzzle, if necessary
- a blanket or beach towel (for warmth)
- a bath towel (can be used as splint)
- a bottle of saline eyewash
- a bottle of artificial tears
- 2 rectal thermometers or digital thermometers
- a pair of bandage scissors
- a pair of tweezers
- a flashlight (with extra batteries)
- a bottle of antihistamine
- a box of baking soda

7

- If your pet is cooperative, you could try making leg bandages or taking his temperature. (It is likely that your dog will be impatient with your unfamiliar manipulations, however; you could practice bandaging on a stuffed animal.)

- Practice lifting and carrying your dog according to the suggestions you will read later on in this book.

- Practice driving the route to your nearest veterinary emergency facility.

- Establish a professional relationship with the clinic and keep emergency telephone numbers handy (for example, in your wallet, in your car and on your refrigerator).

- Review this book periodically to keep basic concepts fresh in your mind.

How to Approach a Frightened or Injured Dog

In a medical emergency, an injured dog that remains conscious will almost certainly be in a state of extreme fear. His anxiety will be further amplified by any pain or disability that he may be experiencing. The animal's natural response will be to try to escape the scene of an accident and to seek shelter in a location where he will feel less vulnerable. Pain and confusion may lead to panic. If he is able to do so, an injured or frightened pet may try to run away if someone approaches, even if that individual is trying to help and even if it is you.

The powerful natural instinct to flee or to stand and fight can be even more pronounced in an injured or sick pet. An injured and panicking dog can easily get lost or worsen his injuries in an attempt to escape from what he perceives to be a menacing person. If the animal feels unable to escape the advance of a potentially harmful person, he may become aggressive, and thus injured or ill animals can be extremely dangerous. These pets must be approached slowly and with great care so as not to aggravate their state of anxiety or to trigger an attack. To approach a dog in an emergency situation (regardless of whether he is obviously afraid):

- Move toward the animal at a steady and very slow pace. Even if the injured or sick dog is your own, avoid the urge to rush to his aid because you could make the situation a lot worse for everyone.

- Keep your arms at your side and avoid sudden movements that could amplify a vulnerable dog's feeling of panic.

- Avoid direct eye contact with the dog. An animal that is in poor physical condition and unable to defend himself may perceive this as an aggressive challenge. Instead, avert your gaze to a point slightly past the animal's shoulder.

> **MAKE AND KEEP REGULAR VETERINARY APPOINTMENTS**
>
> An effective way to prevent a health crisis is to make regular veterinary appointments for your dog. Your veterinarian may discover changes in your dog's health status that you have overlooked. He or she will also keep your dog's vaccinations up-to-date—a critical factor in keeping your dog well.

- Keep your voice soft and soothing. With your calming tone and reassuring words, you may avoid alarming the animal further and he might welcome your approach. Remember that our pets learn to become expert judges of our moods by our body language and verbal intonations. If you project an image of anxiety and panic, the vulnerable animal will become even more defensive.

- If the animal seems to panic increasingly as you come closer, crouch down and stay where you are for a moment. Continue trying to reassure him with your voice before beginning your approach again. If the dog remains agitated or alarmed in any way, it may be necessary to crawl toward him and avoid looking in his direction altogether. Stop your advance every few feet to allow the animal to adjust to your presence.

- If the dog is obviously fearful and aggressive (e.g., showing his teeth in a "lip curl," growling or barking, ears flattened against the head), resist your urge to reach toward him with your hand outstretched over his head. Instead, stay where you are for a few moments longer and remain motionless as you continue talking in a soothing manner. If the dog persists in threatening you, back away to a distance at which he seems to relax or reduce his aggressive displays. Never jeopardize your own safety.

- Some dogs will become more passive when they are leashed. Even if the leash does not help to subdue the dog, you will at least be able to better control his biting end. If possible, get a leash or rope and slowly pass a loop over the animal's head and neck. Once you have secured the leash, the dog may have a change in attitude. Proceed with caution.

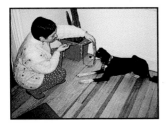

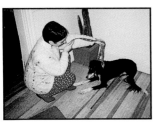

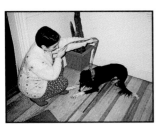

Carefully loop a leash (pass the clip end through the wrist loop end) over the injured dog's head if he is aggressive or if he has no collar. (The author with her Saluki.)

- Another way to approach a dog that does not relax his guard is to use a blanket, sheet or towel as a blind. Open the blanket with your arms held wide so that it covers you but does not quite obstruct your view. When you are close enough, drop the blanket over the injured animal, being sure to cover his head. If he is a small- or medium-sized dog, you may be able to lift him up, being careful to keep the blanket over his eyes and especially his mouth to prevent your being bitten. If he is a large dog, this might give you enough time to move into position to slip a leash around his head as you quickly pull the blanket away.

- In some cases, it may also be necessary to muzzle the dog's mouth to protect yourself as you examine, treat or transport him. If you do not have a dog muzzle, you can use a strip of cloth, panty hose, a soft rope or cord, a long piece of ribbon or a length of gauze bandaging material. Make a loose knot with your material, pass it over the dog's nose and pull the two ends snugly so that the muzzle falls halfway between the dog's nose and eyes. Pass the two ends beneath the dog's chin and tie another knot to secure the mouth. Then bring the two ends under the dog's ears and tie them with a bow (so that it can be easily removed) behind the dog's neck. Muzzle placement may be easier to accomplish once a leash has first been placed around the dog's neck so that you can control the dog's head movements as you approach his mouth. If you are unable to leash the dog, however, a muzzle may also be difficult to place. Most importantly, do not jeopardize your own safety.

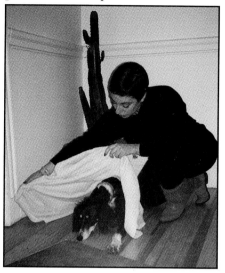

Putting a towel or blanket over a dog that seems disturbed can help.

- If you feel unable to safely approach the victim or even if you simply lack the confidence to offer assistance, get help. Go to the nearest telephone and call a friend, an animal shelter, animal control officer or veterinary clinic for their advice and possible intervention at the scene.

chapter 2

Basics
of
First Aid

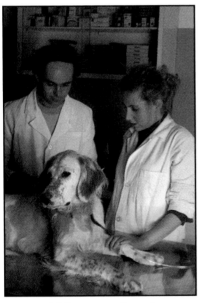

If you think that it might be an emergency, then it is. No one knows better than you do what constitutes an emergency situation. You know your dog's normal habits and behavior, including her moods, facial expressions, bowel and bladder habits and appetite. You should call your veterinary clinic and describe your pet's symptoms with any of your concerns for her well-being. It is always better to err on the side of caution. The hospital staff is trained to recognize when an animal should be seen on an immediate emergency basis, as a fit-in appointment within twenty-four hours or as a regular appointment within several days. If the staff seems to think there is no immediate danger to your pet despite your concern, leave a message to speak with your veterinarian.

In general, you should *seek immediate veterinary care* if your dog:

- has been hit by a car (even without obvious injury),

- has suffered any type of traumatic injury (e.g., dog fight, fallen from heights, sudden lameness),

- has survived, even in the absence of obvious injury, any type of traumatic event (such as being a passenger in a car that was in an automobile accident),

- has lost consciousness even briefly, regardless of the cause,

- is bleeding uncontrollably (even after ice and/or pressure is applied),

- has difficulty walking,

- has difficulty breathing,

- has difficulty urinating (strains or cries when urinating, unable to void urine, or bloody urine),

- has diarrhea with blood.

As a rule, you should make an *appointment for your dog to be seen within twenty-four hours* if your dog:

- seems to be in minor discomfort (e.g., chews at her feet, scratches more than usual, whimpers when she walks or urinates) and/or is behaving unusually (e.g. is socially withdrawn, shows loss of appetite),

- has a recognized medical condition of any kind and is showing physical changes or is behaving unusually,

- is currently on any medication and is showing physical changes or is behaving unusually,

- has a minor traumatic injury that initially responds to your first aid,

- has difficulty seeing (squinting, tearing, discharge, itchiness) from one or both eyes,

- has difficulty defecating (strains or vocalizes when attempting to defecate, absence of stools for more than twenty-four hours, small amount of blood on formed stools) or has diarrhea.

If you have any doubts as to the severity of a problem, have your pet seen on an emergency basis. *Trust your instincts.* Acting quickly may prevent a minor emergency from escalating into a major problem. Perhaps the single most important thing to do to prevent an emergency is to *call your veterinary clinic as soon as you detect a problem with your dog.* Please do not feel that your perception of a potential problem involving your dog is only imaginary or unimportant. One of the greatest frustrations of veterinary practice is being confronted with a problem that the pet has endured for unnecessarily long periods. Some conditions become increasingly difficult to treat even after just a few days are allowed to pass. It is never inappropriate to call and speak to your veterinarian. His or her primary concern, like yours, is the well-being of your pet.

Monitoring Breathing

There are a number of ways to monitor a dog's breathing (respiration). Practice evaluating your dog's normal breathing before an emergency situation arises. It is important to recognize several characteristics that qualify breathing:

FREQUENCY (RESPIRATORY RATE)

Small dogs breathe faster than larger ones and the rate of any dog's breathing will increase after exercise and in times of stress. The normal respiratory rate is between ten and thirty breaths per minute. To evaluate your dog's rate of breathing, watch the rise and fall of your dog's chest. When she inhales, the chest will rise as the lungs fill with air and use the essential oxygen it carries. When she exhales, the chest will fall as air moves out and takes with it carbon dioxide gas that is produced as a by-product of metabolism. When you count the respiratory frequency, count either the number of times your dog inhales (chest rises) or exhales (chest falls) over a sixty-second period. A shortcut is to count the frequency over a thirty-second interval and multiply by two (respirations/minute).

It can be difficult to assess breathing only by sight. In an emergency, respirations may be shallow or even absent (see the discussion of artificial respiration later in this chapter) and can be hard to evaluate in a very heavy dog or a dog with a thick, long coat. Rather than observing the chest movement, place your hand or face within 1 or 2 inches of the dog's nostrils to feel the warm breath as it is exhaled through the nose. Try this with a small mirror and you will see water vapor condense on the mirror's surface as the animal exhales. Another simple technique is to place your hand lightly on the dog's chest over the ribs, midway between her forearm and abdomen, to feel the dog's breathing motions.

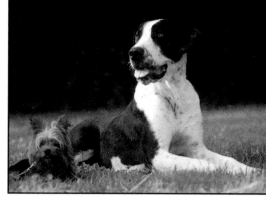

Small dogs breathe more rapidly than larger dogs.

QUALITY

Watch and listen to your dog when she is resting comfortably. In general, normal respiration through the nostrils is almost silent (unless the dog has a short muzzle and small nostrils found in breeds such as the Bulldog or Boston Terrier). In open-mouthed breathing, or panting, the sounds are more audible even in a dog with a standard muzzle. A wheezing sound, however, might indicate a restricted airway. A gurgling sound with each respiration is suggestive of some type of fluid in the respiratory system. In a sick or injured dog, for example, it would be important to report to your veterinarian that the breathing sounded harsh, or heavier than usual, or that there was a yellow or perhaps a bloody discharge from the dog's nostrils.

15

EFFORT

In the well dog, breathing should be an involuntary function. In other words, breathing should be effortless and accomplished unconsciously by the individual.

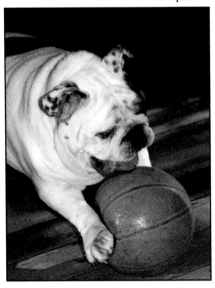

In some emergencies and diseases, breathing is so affected that it is no longer an automatic or painless function. In these cases, breathing is described as "labored" if the pet seems to struggle for breath. Rather than the normal, gentle rise and fall of the chest and ribs with each breath, these movements may appear forced and erratic. The greater the difficulty encountered with each breath, the more likely the dog will pant with her mouth open. The dog's facial expression will reflect her anxiety. In extreme cases, the abdomen appears to pump up and down as the chest heaves with each breath. This is called costoabdominal respiration and is not normal breathing.

Dogs with short muzzles, like Bulldogs, may naturally make noise when they breathe.

Monitoring Heartbeat

The normal canine heart rate (cardiac frequency) ranges between 60 and 160 beats per minute. The wide range of heart rate in dogs depends on a variety of factors, such as the size of the dog, her age, her physical fitness and her emotional state. For example, the heart may beat as fast as 200 beats per minute in young puppies. A healthy adult dog of average size may have a resting heart rate of about 100 beats per minute, but the heart will beat faster if the dog sees another dog, or smells a steak on the barbecue or after she chases a squirrel up a tree. In general, heart rate is directly proportional to the dog's size—smaller dogs tend to have a faster resting heart rate and larger dogs tend to have a slower resting heart rate.

The heart rate will also increase when the body temperature rises due to fever, for example, or when the dog's blood pressure falls due to shock. In a state of medical emergency, a dog may panic or become restless due to pain and the heart rate may rise. Heart rate will decrease in a state of rest, but it can also fall because the animal is ill. Internal hemorrhage, for example, may initially trigger an increase in heart rate as the body tries to stabilize itself; but if it can no longer compensate for a massive drop in blood volume, heart rate may drop. Some diseases, such as hypothyroidism, will also decrease the resting heart rate in dogs.

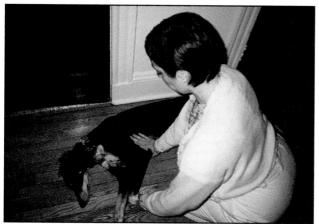

To monitor your dog's heartbeat, bend her left elbow and place your hand on the chest just behind the point of the elbow.

To monitor heart rate, practice on your dog when she is at rest, before an emergency occurs. With the dog lying on her right side, bend the left elbow slightly by lifting up her paw. The elbow will lie just in front of the heart in this position. Rest your hand lightly on the chest wall just behind the left elbow to feel the heart beat. This is the position where the heart muscle comes closest to the body's surface. The heart can be felt on the right side in the same location but not as strongly as on the left side unless the dog is very small, narrow-chested or very young. Ideally, the heart rate should be monitored for a full sixty seconds, but in an emergency this is not always possible. To measure cardiac frequency, count the frequency over a twenty-second interval and multiply by three to obtain the heart rate per minute. Counting over thirty seconds and then multiplying by two, however, may give you a more accurate count. (See the discussion of how to give cardiopulmonary resuscitation at the end of this chapter.)

Signs of Shock

Shock is a physiological phenomenon that results in cardiovascular collapse. Unfortunately, although its function is to defend vital organ systems in an emergency, *a dog can die of the consequences of shock before she succumbs to the effects of her injuries*. Gum color and capillary refill, mental status (alert, sluggish, comatose), heart rate and body temperature are all important reflections of the state of shock.

To evaluate signs of shock, the dog's cardiovascular system must be assessed. This is done by physical examination, which you can do at the scene of an emergency. To evaluate your pet for cardiovascular collapse, one of the basic signs of shock is a slower capillary refill time:

- Lift the side of the dog's mouth to expose the gums; if your pet has pigmented gums (very dark or even black pigment is common in dogs) it may be impractical to assess by this method.

- Gently but firmly press one finger into the gums for one to two seconds (you will notice that the pressure of your finger blocks blood circulation beneath your finger tip so that the gums appear pale) and remove your finger.

- Observe how long it takes for the blanched zone to regain a normal pink color or to return to the same appearance of the gums around it (anything slower than two seconds is a sign of a problem).

Warning: your pet may be in early shock and have normal gum color. Do not dismiss the severity of your dog's condition even if she does not seem in shock to you at the time—take her to the veterinary clinic to be certain that no treatment is necessary. It is most important to note your pet's mental status. If your dog seems sluggish, slow to respond to you or seems lethargic and confused, she should be transported to a clinic *immediately*. If your dog has lost consciousness, do not waste time by examining her for more minor signs of shock.

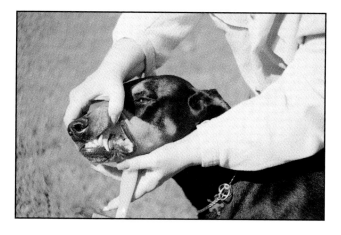

To evaluate your dog for shock, start by lifting her mouth to expose the gums, then pressing on the gums firmly—observe how long it takes for the blanched zone to regain a normal color.

Shock can be caused by many different injuries and diseases but there are common findings. In general, the shock patient will be weak, subdued or even comatose. Her pulse may be rapid and weak. Her body temperature may be below normal but may also be normal or even above normal (for example, in the case of shock secondary to bacterial infection). There are three important categories of medical emergencies resulting in shock:

1. Hypovolemic Shock—anything that causes a reduction of normal blood volume (such as hemorrhage, trauma or dehydration) can lead to this type of shock; gums and other membranes (e.g., inside lining of the eyelids) will be pale and cool.

2. Shock Due to Low Blood Pressure—secondary to central nervous system (brain) disorders or trauma, as well as extreme allergic reactions (anaphylaxis) and drug reactions can result in shock; gums are unusually pink and warm.

3. Shock Due to Infection (Septicemia)—can result from bacterial, viral or fungal infections but can also develop from the other types of shock above;

gums may be blanched but may also appear muddy.

Animals in shock may breathe rapidly but not take deep breaths (hyperventilation). They may be panicked and agitated following an accident. In early stages, the body's defense mechanisms will try to rally to allow an injured or sick dog to escape danger. As these defenses progress, however, signs of shock will become more obvious and extreme, leading to collapse. If your dog is conscious, keep her calm and reassured with your tone of voice. If she is unconscious or seems disoriented following any kind of accident, proceed to your veterinary clinic *immediately*. Cover her with a towel, a blanket or any article of clothing you can spare to maintain her body temperature. If injuries appear superficial or minor (a scratch, for example) yet your dog seems dazed and unable to rise, ignore the scratches and transport her to the clinic *immediately*. If the injury bleeds profusely or if the animal is increasingly lethargic or unconscious, apply first aid to control bleeding and see your veterinarian *immediately*.

If your dog seems disoriented following an accident, cover her with a towel or blanket to maintain her body temperature and take her to the veterinarian immediately.

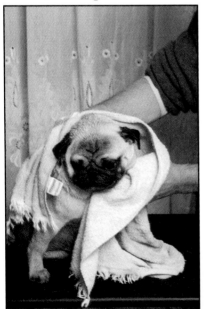

Taking Body Temperature

A dog's normal body temperature is generally between 100 and 103 degrees Fahrenheit (°F) (37.5 to 39.5 °C). The best way to take a measurement of a dog's body temperature is with a rectal thermometer. You may purchase a rectal thermometer at any pharmacy. These are available in the traditional glass version or in digital models. If you drop a glass thermometer, it will shatter and the liquid mercury it contains will spill tiny droplets that can be challenging to retrieve. It also takes about one minute to get an accurate reading. Used with care, the glass thermometer is inexpensive and accurate. Digital models are a bit more costly but give faster readings (within thirty seconds or less) and are fairly accurate. The major disadvantage to relying on a digital thermometer is that the battery may have worn out just when you need to take your pet's temperature. It may be safest to keep one of each type of thermometer (or two of the same type) in your emergency kit and bathroom cabinet, just in case. To measure your dog's temperature:

- Shake the glass thermometer down so that it reads less than 99°F; (this is unnecessary with a digital version). *Note:* In a real emergency, it would be important to shake it down even lower than 99°F, because body temperature can fall to dangerously low levels.

- Lubricate the thermometer tip with a drop of lubricating jelly, petroleum jelly, liquid soap or detergent.

- Gently raise the dog's tail (if your dog has one, that is) so that the anus is exposed. If necessary, part the hair so that you have a clear view of your target.

- Place the thermometer tip against the anus. You may notice that the anal sphincter may tense momentarily, as if it is winking at you.

- When the "winking" slows a bit, gradually insert the thermometer approximately 1 inch into the rectum (approximately one-fourth to one-third of the length of the instrument). Depending on the type of thermometer you use, leave the instrument in for about thirty to sixty seconds. With a glass thermometer, you can watch as the mercury rises for about one minute; when it seems to have stopped, your reading is usually complete. With a digital instrument, you will hear a beep when the measurement is done.

- Slowly withdraw the thermometer and wipe with a tissue or cotton ball. If you are not in an emergency situation, it is also a good idea to disinfect with some soap and water or wipe it again with alcohol before you store it away. In an emergency, you can worry about this detail later!

If you practice with a healthy and alert dog, taking a temperature may be resented so do not insist. This should not be a painful procedure if it is done correctly and with consideration, and it provides vital information regarding your dog's condition. However, *in a life-threatening emergency, taking a body temperature can be skipped in the interest of speeding your dog to an emergency facility.*

Disinfecting Wounds

Wounds at the body surface can be open or closed. Open wounds include cuts (lacerations), scrapes (abrasions), punctures, draining abscesses and open fractures (bone fragments that penetrate the skin to the outside). Closed wounds include bruises (hematoma), closed abscesses, closed fractures and soft tissue injuries such as sprains (joint torsion). These are discussed in more detail elsewhere in this book. Do not attempt to remove an embedded foreign body (debris of any size, knife, wood, metal object) because massive hemorrhage may follow. Instead, keep your dog calm and warm, and proceed *immediately* to the nearest veterinary facility.

Before you disinfect your dog's injuries, examine her more closely. Are there any bones or muscle exposed? If so, the injury is serious and you should proceed to the nearest veterinary facility for treatment. Is your pet becoming agitated or even aggressive when you attempt to examine the wound? Do not risk injury to yourself by trying to disinfect the wound. Leave this to trained professionals.

In many cases, an animal may be injured but the skin is not broken. All you may see is some swelling, pain and perhaps discoloration (deep pink to dark purple) at the injured area. It is generally unnecessary to disinfect this type of injury; the most appropriate thing to do is to apply an ice pack to the swollen area. Whether a wound is open or closed, direct application of ice is almost always helpful and the sooner it is applied, the better. Ice is helpful to minimize swelling (edema), pain and bleeding (hemorrhage). Use an ice pack wrapped in a light cloth or cover the pack with plastic and place it on the wound. Gel-filled flexible ice packs can be purchased at any pharmacy, stored in the freezer and kept ready for use, while chemical ice packs need not be refrigerated and are activated by manipulation. If no ice pack is available, a plastic bag filled with ice cubes is an easy alternative to cover or wrap around the injury. Another option is to use a bag of frozen vegetables (frozen corn or peas work best but any kind will do), which conforms nicely to almost any superficial injury.

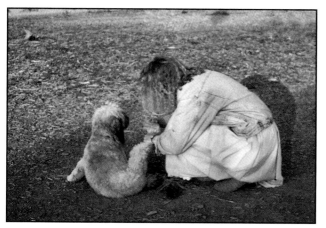

Examine your dog closely before disinfecting an injury. If bones or muscles are exposed, the injury is serious and prompt medical attention is a must.

If an open wound is bleeding, place a sterile gauze pad or a clean cloth over the area and apply direct pressure to the surface. If you have an ice pack, use the ice pack applied with pressure directly to the wound. The combination of pressure and ice causes vessels to constrict and thereby minimizes blood loss. If you do not have an ice pack, direct pressure alone will still be of great benefit.

Bleeding can originate from veins or from arteries of varying sizes. Large amounts of blood can be lost more quickly in arterial hemorrhage (especially if large vessels are damaged) than in hemorrhage from most veins:

23

If the bleeding seems to ooze onto the wound, the bleeding is probably from veins. Do not remove your pressure too soon or any clot that has formed may be torn away and hemorrhage could return.

Arterial bleeding seems to pump in rhythm and this type of bleeding may be more difficult to control. Apply direct pressure and do not remove the pressure for at least five minutes.

If bleeding continues, seek veterinary care *immediately.* In fact, seek veterinary care right away for any open wound whether there is obvious bleeding or not.

If the bleeding wound is small (less than 2 inches or so), apply pressure directly with your fingers (direct manual pressure) and sterile gauze from your emergency kit. You may also use any clean towel or garment. If the wound is larger (greater than 2 inches), you may need to use your whole hand to stop the bleeding.

In general, soap and water remain the best way to clean most minor injuries such as cuts and scrapes. Use a basin of lukewarm water (tap water is acceptable in an emergency, sterile water is best if you have some), a soft face cloth, a sponge or paper towel and a small amount of liquid soap. As a second choice, or as a second step to disinfection, use hydrogen peroxide or betadine (proviodine 1 percent).

Do not rub the wound surface. Gently pour the cleansing solution over the wound directly from the basin or container, or soak a sponge or cloth and squeeze the solution over the area. This will flush away most debris such as bits of gravel, dirt, grass or hair that might be adhering to the wound. If any debris remains even after generous flushing, use a tweezers or even a clean cotton swap to remove as much as you can.

Rinse well with generous amounts of lukewarm water to remove any soap suds or debris that remain on or in the wound. You may apply topical antibiotic (available through your veterinarian or your local pharmacy) to the wound surface. Apply a light dressing until a veterinarian can evaluate the injury.

Avoid touching the wound with your bare hands. By keeping your hands away from the wound, you will not only decrease the risk of infection to your pet, but also protect yourself. Many diseases (such as rabies) are transmitted by direct contact with saliva or blood and you must consider your own safety, particularly when the origin of the wound is unknown or if it was caused by a wild animal or unfamiliar pet of any kind.

It can also be helpful, although not mandatory in an emergency situation, to clip the hair around the wound prior to disinfection so that you can more easily monitor healing. With a scissors sterilized in hot water or rubbing alcohol, carefully trim the hair (to about ⅓ inch in length) about 1 to 2 inches all around the wound. It is not necessary to try to cut the hair very short, as doing so will increase the risk of cutting your dog. If your dog has a smooth, short coat, it is probably not worthwhile to attempt to trim the hair. Your veterinarian uses clipper blades that are specifically intended for use in pets and do not harm the skin.

> ### VACCINATE YOUR DOG AGAINST RABIES
>
> If your pet has been in a fight with another animal or even if you are simply unsure how an open wound was caused, consult with your veterinarian *immediately*. Rabies is reported everywhere in the United States and elsewhere in the world and occasionally epidemics will erupt. Keep your dog's rabies vaccine up-to-date regardless of whether a rabies epidemic is reported in your area (you would not want your dog to be the first reported case in a new outbreak).

Applying Bandages and Splints

For first aid purposes, bandages and splints are intended to be temporary until expert veterinary care is available. Do not feel that your skills need to be perfect.

BANDAGES

Bandages are needed:

1. to cover open wounds to prevent further contamination during transport to the veterinary clinic,
2. to cover bleeding wounds while pressure is applied to control blood loss during transport to the veterinary clinic,

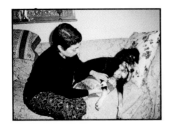

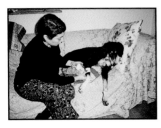

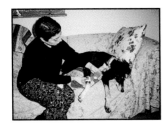

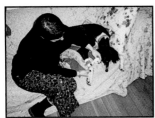

After disinfecting the wound, apply layers of gauze dressing, rolled gauze, bandaging and adhesive tape (do not pull tightly as you wrap or blood circulation may be impaired and cause pain and swelling).

3. to apply slight pressure to an injury to minimize swelling and the sensation of pain before (and after) treatment by a veterinarian,

4. to prevent the dog from creating further harm by licking her own wounds before or after she has received veterinary care,

5. to keep healing wounds clean and dry following veterinary care.

Flush away surface debris and disinfect before applying any bandage to an open wound. This may not always be possible, or even necessary, in an emergency (in the case of a hemorrhaging wound, for example). Apply a square gauze or a sterile nonstick pad large enough to cover the surface wound; if you only have small gauze pads, use several and overlap them to cover the wound; apply several layers to provide a thick dressing for protection and additional absorption. With one hand, hold the dressing to the wound and place the end of the roll of bandaging material across the dressing. Rolled gauze is the preferred material for use as the layer over the local dressing, but if you do not have rolled gauze you may use whatever bandage supplies you have.

Wrap the rolled bandage around the dressing, overlapping by about two-thirds of the width of the bandage material; extend the bandage 1 to 2 inches above and below the edges of the dressing. Do not pull on the bandaging material as you unravel it or the bandage will be too tight (you should be able to easily pass your finger under the edge of the bandage).

If your intent is to apply a pressure bandage to control swelling or bleeding, create a bandage of many layers (use cotton batting in a roll for best results) so that the thickness of the bandage, not the tension, provides the desired pressure.

Use adhesive tape (preferably bandage or surgical tape) to secure the end of the bandage; if you will also be applying additional layers of bandage material (e.g., elastic bandage), it is unnecessary to tape the gauze wrap. If you have an elastic bandage available, apply it loosely, overlapping edges two-thirds of the width of the bandage; cover the inside layers of gauze and extend it about 1 inch beyond the edges of the gauze layer. Secure the end with tape or safety pins (many bandages, available at your local pharmacy, now come with fasteners or are self-adhesive). Use surgical or adhesive tape to cover the top inch of the bandage and 1 inch above the top of the bandage (this is the key to keeping the bandage in place—the adhesive tape must stick to hair or skin so that it will not slip—repeat application of the adhesive tape on the bottom edge of the bandage.

Whenever possible, call ahead to warn the veterinary team that you are on the way with an injured dog; remain calm and proceed directly to the clinic.

SPLINTS

Splints are recommended if there is an obvious or suspected closed fracture, an open fracture or a large gaping wound of a limb. Do not touch any open wound with your bare hands.

An open fracture is one in which the bone fragments protrude at the skin surface. If there is an open fracture or wound, flush debris from the surface (see "Disinfecting Wounds," above), place a clean dressing and, if possible, cover with a sterile dressing and light bandage before splinting the leg. If the wound is bleeding profusely, an ice pack can be bandaged around the site of hemorrhage and the limb immobilized with a splint.

A closed fracture should be suspected if your dog has pain and difficulty in attempts to walk using the injured leg. The fractured limb may be dragged, held off the ground, or simply held in awkward positions so that it does not bear the dog's weight. Some types of fractures are stable—the bone fragments are still held together (like pieces of a jigsaw, they interlock but are not solidly in place) and the dog gingerly may bear weight on the limb. In general, however, the pain of broken bones will deter voluntary movement of the limb. (It should be noted that some severe sprains and other soft tissue injuries can be painful enough initially to disable the limb.)

Although splints are helpful, they should be considered optional first aid. If the dog is able to bear weight on the leg or to control the injured limb (even if it is only to hold it flexed closer to the body) it is probably not worthwhile to make a splint. It would be helpful, with the severe injuries described above, to place a splint on a dog's leg if your dog allows you to do so! Moreover, a splint can help to minimize pain, bone displacement or other complications while you transport your dog for medical treatment. However, it is simply not worth wasting time if your pet panics, is very agitated or becomes aggressive while you try to fabricate a splint and maneuver her injured leg. Under these circumstances, proceed directly to the clinic. Call ahead, if possible, to let them know you will be arriving shortly with an emergency lameness. Open fractures rank high in the list of urgent injuries and should be seen by your veterinarian *immediately*.

For the purposes of first aid, splints are intended as temporary bindings to stabilize an injury during transport. Splints are meant to immobilize an injured limb to minimize aggravation of the injury and pain, and to provide support and cushioning. The splint can be made of improvised materials and secured with any type of adhesive tape, safety pins, belt, string, ribbon, bandaging material or anything else you have available. Some common objects that can be used for splints include:

- A towel—fold the towel in half and, depending on the size of the towel and the size of the dog's leg, in half again; slide the folded towel under the leg and wrap it around toward the top of the leg (it need not encircle the leg entirely). Or, wrap the folded towel snugly but not tightly around the injured limb and secure it in place; it may be most comfortable simply to place the folded towel beneath the injured limb to provide support during transport.

- Any folded garment—the garment can be used as bandaging material to provide a bulky wrap or it can be folded and secured in the same way as the towel, above.

- A newspaper or magazine—a newspaper or magazine can be folded to provide a groove in which to rest the injured leg or it can be shaped into a roll and wrapped around the limb.

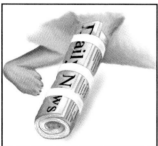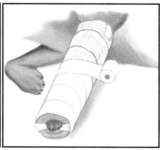

Make a temporary splint by wrapping the leg in a folded newspaper or magazine and securing it by bandaging it.

- Sticks—sticks can be tied directly to the length of the leg for short periods or to provide additional support for bandages.

- Tennis/handball/racquetball/badminton rackets— rackets can provide relatively comfortable and lightweight support. Stringed racquets are, in addition, relatively easy to tie around the limb (just pass string or other binding through the strings!).

- Boards/cardboards—almost any type of board (paper, wood, plastic, metal) can be used to support an injured limb as long as there are no sharp edges or splinters!

- Cardboard rolls from paper toweling (cardboard rolls from toilet paper for small dogs and puppies)— the injured leg can be passed inside the roll and then a towel or cloth wrapped around; the cardboard roll can be cut lengthwise to be more easily contoured to the leg and secured with tape.

How to Lift, Carry and Transport an Injured Dog

There are many methods of lifting an injured animal. You will need to consider the location of the emergency (e.g., in a ditch, in your yard, in a lake) in addition to the nature of your dog's injuries (unconscious, broken leg, bleeding wound). The size of the dog and her temperament are also important factors that will affect how she may be carried. Before you attempt to lift any dog, be sure that you understand the suggestions for how to approach a frightened/injured dog set forth in chapter 1. Always remember to protect yourself from injury. You cannot help your dog if you are hurt in an attempt to rescue your cherished companion.

If your dog is able to walk but has an injured limb or other obvious injury, you may need to lift and carry her to your vehicle. Regardless of whether your dog is able to walk, avoid bending her body or making abrupt movements. Some injuries are undetectable at the accident scene. The method of lifting your dog will depend greatly on her size and the extent of her injuries:

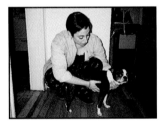

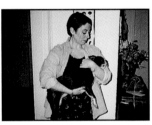

To lift a small dog, hold her head and neck against you as you lift her under her belly and chest.

- To lift a small dog (less than 30 pounds), slowly and gently place one arm along the length of her abdomen and chest and cradle her body close to yours. With your other hand, hold your dog's head and neck close to you to prevent her from turning to snap at you as well as to give her a sense of security in your arms.

- To lift a medium-sized dog, hug your dog's neck into the crook of your elbow and gently draw her head into your body. Pass your other arm under her abdomen just in front of her legs and reach upward toward her back as you cradle her body to yours. Another way to lift is to wrap your arm around the front of her chest just above the front legs and your other arm under her belly. Use your legs, not your back, to lift a medium- or large-sized dog. It is also helpful to exhale (holding your breath may predispose you to injury) as you stand and lift your precious cargo.

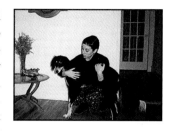

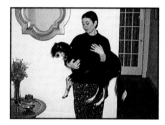

- To lift a large dog, you can hug her head and neck as described above, but it may be more comfortable to wrap your arm around the front of her chest just above the front legs or under her chest. Pass your other arm under her rump just above the back of the knees. Again, it is very important to keep your back straight, exhale gradually and use your leg muscles to stand.

To lift a medium-sized dog, wrap one arm around the front of her chest just above the front legs and lift under her belly.

If someone is available to help you lift your medium- or large-sized dog, the same techniques apply. It is recommended that you stay at your dog's head and have your assistant lift the rear end. Synchronize the lift by counting out loud to two or three. Reassure your dog as you lift and carry her. She may struggle to get free because of pain or panic. Keep your hold firm but do not grip tightly unless it is absolutely necessary to prevent further injury to yourself or your pet.

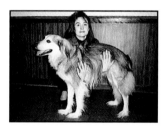

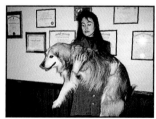

To lift a large dog, pass one arm under her chest just behind the front legs and the other under her rear behind the knees—lift with your legs and not your back.

If your dog is unconscious or unable to walk, she may be suffering from serious internal injuries or head and spinal cord trauma. For these patients, (and for a large- or giant-sized dog that is too heavy to lift) it might be best to transport on a stretcher. For small- and medium-sized patients, you

31

can use a box or even an open suitcase. If a piece of plywood or particle board is available, you could lift this alone, but it would be better with the help of an assistant. You may also use the lid of a garbage can, a sled or a toboggan. If you have enough time, tie a rope or belt around your dog to secure her to the board at the level of her shoulder and hip. Remember that the stretcher has to fit into the car, so it may only be of use to transport the dog to the vehicle. If you are at home, you might use an ironing board to carry your pet, but these are narrow and you must keep your patient balanced, even if she is secured to the board. If you are unable to easily locate an item that could be used as stretcher, don't waste time constructing a makeshift stretcher. It is far more important to get your dog to the nearest emergency facility as quickly as possible. More often than not, the easiest and best stretcher will be a jacket or coat, blanket or sheet, mat or area rug. Cover your injured dog with a blanket or any article of clothing to preserve body heat. Place your dog's back against the back of the car seat or even on the floor of your vehicle so that it will not be unnecessarily jostled during transport. Your pet already has enough problems without rolling off the car seat.

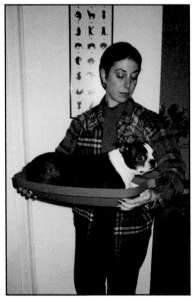

Almost anything can be used as a stretcher—for a small dog, a garbage can lid will work just fine.

Drive carefully! Concentrate on traffic, road obstacles and the shortest route to your destination. Obviously, successful transportation of the patient to the emergency facility is a critical aspect of first aid. Don't forget to breathe! Continue speaking to your dog in a calm and soothing voice while you drive.

How to Give Medication

Medicating a sick or injured dog can be one of the greatest challenges of pet ownership. Somehow, even the most passive and eager to please dog can become downright ornery when it comes to being medicated or manipulated in order to receive medication. The administration of prescribed drugs can be important in preventing emergencies. For example, your dog may be on a course of prescribed drugs to treat a serious illness. Although the administration of medication will rarely be required of the dog owner in an emergency, you might be instructed to do so by your veterinarian.

Never administer any kind of medication or treatment to your dog without first consulting with your veterinarian. Do not assume that a remedy that has been recommended in the past for a particular symptom will again be appropriate should the same or similar symptoms recur. Many medical conditions resemble one another, but their treatments may be very different. An accurate diagnosis must be made and you should not guess at what treatment is right for your pet without your veterinarian's input.

HOW TO GIVE ORAL MEDICATION

Medicines that are to be taken by mouth (oral) come in tablet (chewable or non chewable), capsule, gel capsule and liquid forms.

To administer medication in pill form directly into the dog's mouth:

1. Place your dog in a "sit" or "down-stay" position. It will be helpful if her back is against the wall. For smaller dogs, place them in your lap or atop an elevated surface.

2. Wrap your thumb and fingers over the top of the dog's muzzle and slide them down toward the mouth; slide your fingers over the lips and draw the lips over the teeth and slightly inside the mouth (this way if your dog bites down or tries to close her mouth she will nip her own lips and not your fingers!).

3. Gently elevate the head with the same hand that is holding the mouth open. Do not raise the head

too far back or the ability to swallow could be affected.

4. With your other hand, drop the tablet or capsule to the very back of the tongue so that the medication is more likely to be swallowed.

5. Release the dog's muzzle and gently hold the mouth closed with your fingers. To encourage swallowing, gently rub her nose with a finger (she will swallow and try to lick her nose) or blow gently onto her nose to tickle it (this will also stimulate swallowing and licking her nose). Rubbing her throat may also be effective to trigger the swallowing reflex.

6. Watch your dog for a few moments after you release her mouth. Some animals can become very adept at holding onto a pill without swallowing it. Be sure the medication is introduced far back on the tongue so that this trick is less successful.

To give a tablet or capsule, it is generally not recommended to crush the medicine in food. Most drugs

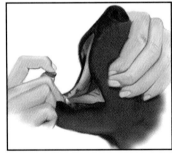

To give a pill, open the mouth wide, then drop it in the back of the throat.

have an unpleasant taste and this will be released when the tablet is crushed or the capsule coating is unsealed.

If you are unable to give a pill directly into your dog's mouth by the method described above, you may need to hide it in food or a treat. Always be sure that the tablet or capsule has been swallowed. Your dog might eat around the pill and leave it in her dish or carry the pill elsewhere and then spit it out. For that reason it is preferred to hide the medication in a small portion of food (a piece of soft cheese, peanut butter, luncheon meat, a piece of hot dog or any favorite food item that is just large enough to cover the pill) and stay to watch as your dog consumes the treat and its hidden "cargo."

Another method is to fill an ice cube tray with chicken or beef broth that has been cooled; place the dose of medication in each compartment and freeze immediately. Now your dog has a special treat that also hides the medication (pill form or liquid) effectively.

For smaller dogs, place a small spoon of broth or water along with the measured medication into the freezer; allow the spoonful of frozen medicated treat to thaw just enough to slide off the spoon before giving it to your pet to enjoy! For very small dogs or for those that do not enjoy frozen treats, freeze the pills in a $\frac{1}{4}$ or $\frac{1}{2}$ teaspoon of water; these will slide easily over the tongue and be swallowed without being tasted at all!

Some solid oral medications are prepared as chewable tablets that are specially flavored to appeal to your dog. Most dogs find these tablets very palatable but, if your dog refuses them, mix the chewable tablet with the dog's food or favorite treat as discussed above.

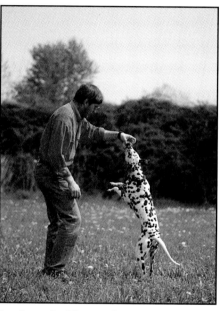

To administer liquid oral medication, gently place the spoon or dropper at the corner of the dog's mouth where the top and bottom lips meet. Deliver the liquid onto the back of the tongue by placing the tip of the spoon or dropper between the back teeth. If your dog resents the flavor of the liquid medication (spits up, drools heavily or foams at the mouth) you could try mixing it into her food or hiding it in a special food treat or frozen treat as described above.

It is preferred to hide medication in a treat—make sure that your dog has swallowed the pill.

Avoid giving oral medication far back in the throat with the head elevated in line with the neck. This posture increases the risk of aspirating the liquid or tablet (inhaling into the lungs). A 45° angle of elevation is safe, effective and need not be exceeded.

If your veterinarian has instructed you to remove food and/or water from your dog, do not administer medication in food treats as described above unless you consult with your dog's veterinarian.

If you have difficulty medicating your dog despite great efforts, do not hesitate to seek help from someone at your veterinary clinic. Gadgets commonly known as "pill poppers" are available through your veterinarian and can be very helpful. Unfortunately, some dogs can be very determined and refuse any attempt to be medicated or treated. In fact, some can become aggressive or unintentionally injure their owners during attempts to treat them. In this case, you may be required to bring your pet to the clinic for her daily treatment, or an alternative medication or route of administration (e.g., injectable) may be advised. It might be necessary to hospitalize or board your dog at the clinic until all the necessary treatments have been completed.

KEEPING CALM WILL SOOTHE YOUR DOG

If your dog is injured but still able to walk, leash her to restrain her from running away and to help keep her subdued. Keep calm and speak softly to your dog to reassure her. Even if a dog does not seem badly injured, she may be in a state of high anxiety and have as yet inconspicuous symptoms of shock. Avoid making sudden movements or rushing toward your dog. Instead, keep your arms relaxed and your facial expression as neutral as possible. Your dog is always attuned to your verbal cues, facial expressions and body language and will be even more responsive in a crisis. You would not want your dog to mistake your concern for impending punishment, nor would you want to amplify your dog's anxiety by panicking yourself.

HOW TO GIVE EYE MEDICATION

Eye (ophthalmic) medications come in liquid or ointment form. Eye drops may be slightly easier to apply than ointments because they can be delivered more quickly. However, some dogs feel uncomfortable when they feel the drop fall onto the surface of the eye. Ointments may take a bit more control to deliver to the eye but may, in some instances, remain in the eye longer for greater benefit in healing. Discuss the advantages and disadvantages of a liquid or ointment ophthalmic medication with your veterinarian in case the drug he or she has chosen is available in both forms. Ask someone at home to help hold your dog if she squirms or resists your attempts to medicate her eyes.

To administer ophthalmic drops/ointment to your dog:

1. Slide the skin of the upper eyelid towards the top of the head; your dog will naturally move her eye downward and away from you as you steady her head with the side of your palm.

2. With your other hand, hold the medication bottle or tube and rest the side of your palm on the side of your dog's face just off to the side of the eye being medicated (this will also help to steady the dog's face to minimize further injury to the eye in case she struggles).

3. Instill the required number of drops or the recommended amount of ointment onto the outside corner of the eye's surface and release the upper eyelid as you allow the eyelids to gently blink.

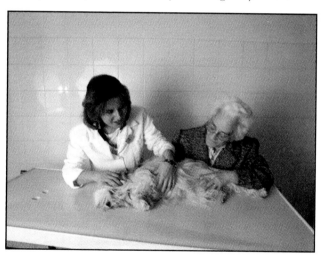

If your dog refuses to be medicated you may need to bring her to the veterinary clinic for treatment.

You may want to give your dog a pea-sized treat as a reward for her tolerance of your manipulation. A treat might increase her patience with you when the next treatment is due!

How to Give Ear Medication

Ear (otic) medication is available in liquid and ointment form. Your veterinarian will prescribe the medication that is appropriate for your dog's ear problem. An ear culture may be necessary, but might not be suggested unless your dog's ears do not respond to the first medication selected for use. Treatments might be easier if you place your dog in a controlled position with her back to the wall or, for smaller dogs, on your lap or a chair.

Lift the ear to view the ear's internal structures and to visualize the entrance to the ear canal.

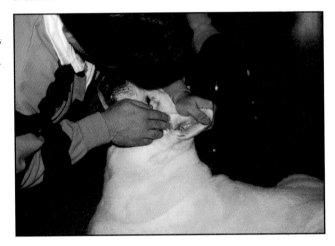

To administer otic medication to your dog:

1. Lift the external part of the ear, if necessary, to view the internal structures of the ear and, most importantly, to visualize the entrance to the ear canal. Most ear infections originate deep inside the ear canal and medication must be instilled directly into the canal to be effective.

2. Gently place the nozzle of the tube or bottle as deep as possible into the canal (these containers are designed to deliver otic medications into the dog's ear canal) and instill the recommended dosage of medication. You will not injure your dog's ear because the canal turns at a right angle and the container tip cannot reach the ear drum.

3. Gently massage the base of your dog's ear to help distribute the medication inside the ear canal.

If your dog is not on a rigid diet, give her a tiny but tasty treat as a reward for her patience and tolerance of your manipulation. It may facilitate the next treatment!

How to Give CPR

Cardiopulmonary resuscitation (CPR) is the popular name given to two distinct emergency procedures: 1) artificial respiration, which allows oxygen to be delivered when breathing has stopped, and 2) heart massage (cardiac massage), which maintains blood flow when the heart has ceased to beat on its own. In many cases, breathing and heartbeat will stop together and both artificial respiration as well as heart massage will be necessary, but this is not always so. Sometimes, the heart will continue to beat (for a few minutes) even when respiration has stopped and breathing may continue briefly when the heart has arrested. It is, therefore, important to determine three things before CPR is attempted:

1. Make sure that the patient is unconscious. You do not want to perform CPR on an animal that does not need it or that might bite you if you try to breathe into her nose unnecessarily; call the dog's name loudly, clap your hands above her head, rub your knuckles across her ribs, pinch (hard if necessary) the skin between the toes to see if she pulls her paw away. If the dog responds to any of the above, delay performing CPR.

2. Verify the presence or absence of a heartbeat. The beating heart will be felt most strongly on the left side of the chest just behind the bent elbow but can also be detected on the right side of the chest. Place your palm over the dog's chest and press down slightly for better contact with the heartbeat (this will be especially important with dogs that have a thick coat or are very overweight). You may also verify the capillary refill of the gums (see p.18) or check for a pulse in the neck (carotid artery) or inside the leg (femoral artery), but feeling the dog's chest is a far more reliable test in an emergency.

3. Verify the presence or absence of breathing. Watch for even a faint movement of the ribs (place your hands lightly on the dog's chest wall if you are

unsure of what you see). Put your hands just in front of the nostrils to detect warm air as it is expelled.

Note: If artificial respiration, cardiac massage or both are required, call for help and transport your dog *immediately* to the nearest veterinary clinic. If possible, call ahead to notify the veterinary staff of the nature of your emergency and approximately when you will arrive.

To give artificial respiration:

1. Make sure that the dog is unconscious and not breathing, as described above.

2. Place the dog on her right side. Should you need to administer cardiac massage, the left side of the chest will already be accessible—an important exception to this is when there is an obvious chest wound on the left side. In this case, place the dog on her left side (despite the injury) so that the healthy lung on the right side is free to breathe more easily.

3. Examine the mouth and back of the throat to remove any foreign matter that could be blocking the airway or that might fall into the airway when you begin artificial respiration. If the unconscious dog is not breathing and her chest does not inflate when you begin artificial respiration, check the inside of the mouth and throat. Open the mouth by parting the upper and lower jaws, and pull the tip of the tongue forward and downward toward the dog's chest to dislodge any obstructing material and to get a clear view; remove solid debris and wipe away any heavy mucus, saliva, blood, vomit or foreign object that may be found. If necessary, reach with your fingers into the back of the dog's throat to feel for any obstructing object or material. If you see an object but cannot reach it, use a spoon or tweezers (do not to push it further into the airway!); administer CPR *immediately following* removal of the obstruction.

4. Encircle the dog's muzzle with one hand and support her neck with your other hand (avoid unnatural neck positions that could interfere with the flow of air or aggravate any hidden injury).

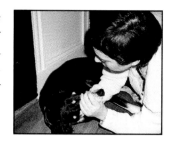

5. Keeping the mouth closed firmly, place your mouth over the dog's nose and exhale deeply enough (but without force) to bring about a moderate rise of the patient's rib cage, signaling adequate inflation of the lungs.

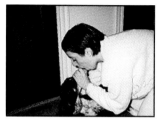

6. Remove your mouth from the dog's nose to allow the lungs to deflate and the dog to exhale. (Do not let go of the muzzle; keep your face close to the dog for efficient technique but your eyes on the patient's chest to monitor the rise and fall of the rib cage and lungs.)

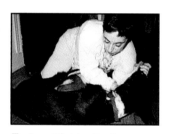

7. Repeat each assisted breath every three to five seconds.

8. Check for the presence of a heartbeat at least three times every minute by placing one hand on the chest wall just behind the dog's bent left elbow. If there is no heartbeat, you will need to begin heart massage as described below. To avoid permanent brain injury, do not stop artificial respiration for longer than thirty seconds; continue CPR during transport as needed.

To give artificial respiration, 1) hold the dog's muzzle and support the neck, 2) exhale into the dog's nose and 3) watch the rise and fall of the dog's chest.

Note: If the dog's gum color does not return to a more normal pink, or if the chest does not rise or fall when you perform artificial respiration, the airway may be obstructed. Try to lift the dog's hind quarters in an effort to expel whatever solid or liquid matter might be obstructing the flow of air; suspend the dog for about five seconds and if possible, have someone compress the middle of each side of her chest. Check the mouth and throat again to remove or wipe away anything that has been expelled and return to artificial respiration. The chances of reviving the dog are, unfortunately, very remote if the airway is obstructed.

If the dog coughs or seems to move in any way, suspend your CPR and check to see if she has begun to breathe independently and if a heartbeat is present. *Do not continue CPR if the dog is breathing and the heart is beating.* Observe your patient for any changes in case you need to resume resuscitation and transport her to the nearest veterinary clinic *immediately*.

To give cardiac massage:

1. Place the dog on her right side, with the left side facing up, as the base of the heart is closest to the surface in this position. If the dog has an obvious injury to the right side of the chest, place the dog on her left side (cardiac massage might be a bit less efficient to the right side of the chest but you need not risk puncturing a lung or the heart with broken ribs during CPR!).

    An alternative position for deep-chested large dogs, very obese dogs or those with obvious chest injuries requires the dog to be placed slightly on her back; place one hand on either side of the dog's chest about one-third of the way between the sternum and the elbow; compress the chest between both your hands (see below).

2. If possible, elevate the dog's hips to facilitate the flow of blood returning to the brain and vital organs.

3. Place one hand over the other just behind and slightly below the bent elbow, interlocking fingers for greater stability; use one hand for small breeds and young puppies.

4. With firm, downward plunges, compress the chest wall over the heart and release between each compression (without removing your hands) at a rate of 100 to 120 compressions per minute (count out loud to help keep the rhythm: "1-and-2-and-3-and-4-and-5-and-1-and-2-and-3-and-4-and-10-and-1-and-2-and-

3-and-4-and-15:" compress on each digit, release on "and"). Do not worry about pressing too hard, but on the other hand avoid compressing the chest too roughly; think of the action of jumping up and down on a trampoline . . .

5. If you are alone and both artificial resuscitation and cardiac massage are required (unassisted CPR), perform two quick breaths after every fifteen cardiac compressions.

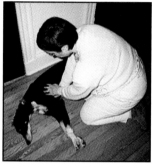

If you have an assistant, one person should perform artificial resuscitation and the other should perform cardiac massage; synchronize your efforts at a rate of one breath per three to five compressions.

Stop CPR every three to five minutes (or before if any movement is detected) to check for the presence of a pulse or heartbeat and for independent respiration. If the dog's pupils remain fixed and dilated despite CPR, a good prognosis (final outcome) is unlikely.

Cardiac massage is performed by overlapping both hands over the heart just behind the dog's left elbow.

As mentioned above, do not stop artificial respiration for longer than thirty seconds to avoid permanent brain injury; continue performing CPR during transport as needed.

Note: If artificial respiration and/or cardiac massage is required, call for help and transport your pet *immediately* to the nearest veterinary clinic. Call ahead, whenever possible, to notify the veterinary staff of the nature of your emergency and approximately when you will arrive.

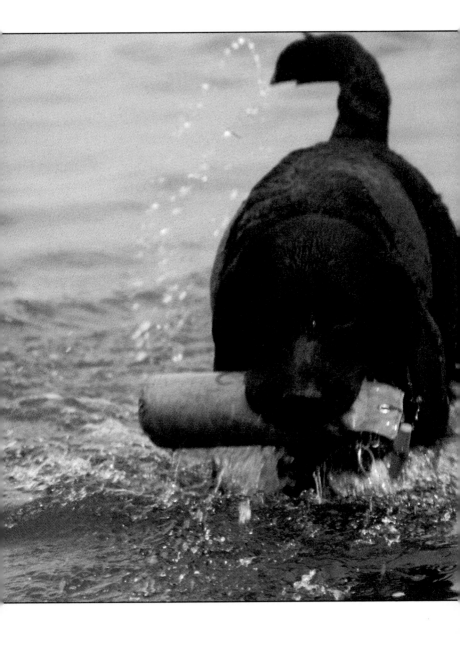

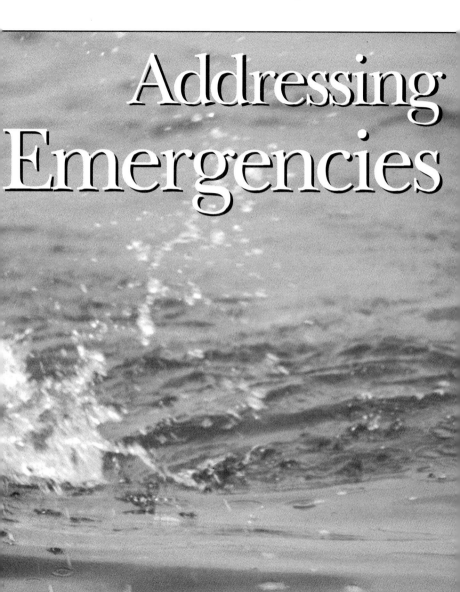

part two

Addressing
Emergencies

chapter 3

External
Wounds

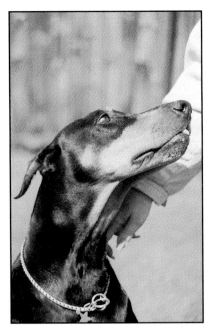

External problems in your dog can range from chewing gum stuck to his foot to a nasty bite from another dog. Regardless of the problem's severity, you will want to address it quickly and properly.

Abscesses

If you find a local swelling of any size on your dog, it could be an abscess, but it could also be a tumor, cyst, insect bite, hematoma (pocket of blood caused by blunt trauma), fracture or soft tissue trauma (sprain, pocket of fluid). To distinguish these maladies from an abscess, you should know that:

- an abscess will usually be warm or even hot to the touch,

- touching the swelling may be painful to the dog (be careful not to antagonize an injured dog),

- your dog may have an elevated body temperature (103° or higher) or he may have a normal temperature,

- your dog may withdraw socially and stop eating or he may behave normally in every way,

- breaks in the skin (bite, scratch, puncture, insect stinger and the like) near or at the swelling site usually indicate the route of bacterial invasion,

- a maturing abscess that is close to rupturing will have a softer spot (or several areas of uneven consistency) where surface rupture is likely,

- recent conflict with another animal increases the likelihood that the swelling is an abscess even if an injury is unnoticeable at first.

An abscess can occur anywhere on the body. Sometimes, the source of the infection is not external (from an injury) but internal (from inside the body). The most common example is from a tooth root abscess of the upper row of teeth that produces a characteristic abscess on the cheek below the eye. The treatment for a tooth root abscess includes draining the abscess, appropriate antibiotics and dental extraction by your veterinarian. The anal glands or sacs, scent-marking organs located on either side of the anus, can become impacted and infected. Infected anal glands (anal sacculitis) can rupture at or near the anus and are painful and sometimes complicated to heal. Anal glands should be examined by your veterinarian if your dog is chewing at his backside, scooting his rump along the ground, biting at his tail or seems to be uncomfortable when you approach his tail. Some dogs never have problems with anal glands while others have ongoing difficulties that can require surgical excision of the infected sacs.

If your pet has a swelling on his body surface that might be an abscess, you should schedule a veterinary visit within twenty-four hours. In the interim, an ice pack placed at the site may provide some relief. Take the dog's rectal temperature to make sure that it is normal. If the temperature is elevated, your veterinarian will want to see your dog the same day to expedite treatment. If your pet has a fever, do not give any aspirin or other medication that might mask the fever. The fever response is an adaptive defense mechanism that benefits your dog and, in most cases, you should not interfere. The problem is not the fever—the problem is the infection. Do not feed your dog the day of your veterinary visit in case he requires surgical drainage on the same day. Any wound infested with maggots (fly larvae) should receive immediate attention. These immature insects burrow deep into the dog's skin and create complicated wounds and much misery. Please do not delay veterinary attention.

If your dog is chewing at his backside, biting at his tail or scooting his rump along the ground, he may have infected anal glands.

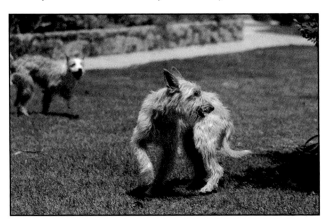

If the abscess has already begun to drain pus:

- do not touch it with your bare hands! Put on latex exam gloves, dish-washing gloves or any type of glove that you can wash later,

- if your dog tolerates it and if you have the stomach for it, wipe the pus away with a paper towel, and press gently on the abscess to encourage further drainage from the open wound,

- pour lukewarm water into the wound to flush out additional infected material and debris,

- additional flushing with hydrogen peroxide may be helpful, once most of the pus is out of the cavity of the abscess,

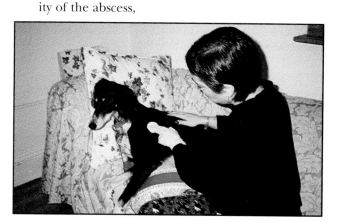

Wear plastic gloves when treating infected wounds or sores.

- cover with a clean dressing and secure with a bandage (see chapter 2),

- call your veterinarian for an appointment *the same day.*

Laceration

A laceration is a cut. Lacerations can be minor and superficial or they can be deep and severe. Superficial cuts can bleed profusely and long gaping wounds can produce minimal bleeding. Refer to the discussions in chapter 2 on disinfecting wounds, making a bandage and bleeding for additional details.

If the cut is superficial and relatively small (less than 1 inch long), cover the wound with a clean or sterile gauze or paper towel and apply direct manual pressure for at least five minutes to stop the bleeding; ideally, place an ice pack over the dressing and apply direct manual pressure. If the bleeding continues when you release pressure, resume

---

WOUNDS OF UNKNOWN ORIGIN

If you do not know how your pet was originally wounded or if it was due to contact with another animal of any kind, there is a small but significant risk of contact with the rabies virus. This virus causes a fatal disease in all mammals, including people, and is transmitted through contact with any bodily fluid. Avoid direct contact with any open wound and seek veterinary attention for your dog without delay. In addition to any treatments necessary for the wound, a rabies vaccination booster may be necessary (even if your dog has had one recently) and your veterinarian will advise you on any quarantine period that is required by law in your area. Keep all your pet's vaccinations, including the rabies vaccine, current throughout his lifetime.

pressure for an additional five to ten minutes before releasing. Sprinkle about 1 teaspoon of sodium bicarbonate onto the wound and continue to apply direct pressure (with ice). If a small cut continues bleeding for more than fifteen minutes, call your veterinarian to be seen right away.

If bleeding has stopped or was never significant, pour soapy, lukewarm water over the wound and follow with clear lukewarm water to flush away any superficial debris. Pat or blot dry; rubbing the surface may disturb blood clots and bleeding could resume. Apply a topical antibiotic ointment (from your first aid kit) and apply a bandage or light dressing. Keep the bandage clean and dry and change the bandage and dressing on a daily basis. If the wound seems to be clean and dry, simply reapply the ointment. However, if you see any sign of redness surrounding the cut or any discharge resembling pus, or if the wound remains open after several days, flush with hydrogen peroxide and pat dry before reapplying the ointment and dressing. If there is no improvement after three to five days, or if the wound causes the animal pain or a fever develops, you should schedule a veterinary visit as soon as possible for additional treatment.

If the wound is greater than 1 inch long and cuts deeply into the skin's layers or deeper still into subcutaneous or muscular layers, cover the wound with a clean or sterile gauze, paper towel or towel and apply direct pressure to stop the bleeding. Use an ice pack to complement the effects of manual pressure; do not release your pressure for a full ten minutes. Gently pour soapy, lukewarm water over the wound and follow with clear lukewarm water to flush away any superficial debris (do not rub the surface—pat it dry). Apply a bandage or light dressing and call the veterinary hospital to advise them that you are on the way in with an emergency laceration.

If a laceration bleeds profusely around your hands during manual pressure and shows no sign of slowing down after five minutes, *do not release your pressure. Note:* bleeding from the ears, feet or tail is often messy and although these injuries require professional care they are not fatal; uncontrolled bleeding elsewhere deserves immediate veterinary attention. Transport your dog to the nearest clinic *immediately*.

If the wound is on the tail or a limb, try applying direct manual pressure to the major supply vessels closer to the body (elevate the tail/limb if possible):

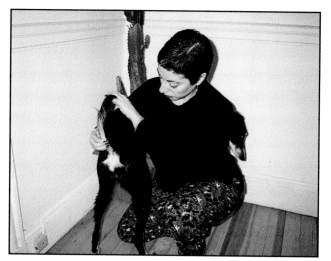

If your dog wounds his tail, apply direct pressure to the tail's major blood supply vessels, located under the tail in the midline groove, to control heavier bleeding.

- Tail—press your fingers along the midline groove that runs the length of the tail to compress the major supply vessels.

- Front leg—wrap your hand around the leg and squeeze tightly about halfway to the shoulder or just above the elbow (depending on where the cut is located and which seems to help more).

- Rear leg—wrap your hand around the lower leg and squeeze tightly if the injury is below this level; for leg injuries above the knee, major supply vessels are located on the inside of the thigh about one-third of the way between the front and back of the leg; apply pressure to the inside of the leg with flattened fingers.

If the wound is on a tail or limb and direct manual pressure to the major vessels fails, apply a tourniquet (discussed below) above the laceration site; gradually

51

tighten the tourniquet until bleeding stops or at least slows down. Tourniquets are a last resort and can cause permanent injury if left on for too long, but in an emergency, the risk is worthwhile. Transport your dog *immediately* to the nearest veterinary facility. Remain calm and keep your pet calm to minimize further blood loss.

If a laceration of any size starts to bleed again despite your efforts, resume direct pressure with any clean dressing or towel and proceed directly to the nearest veterinary facility.

For a rear leg injury, apply direct manual pressure to the large vessels of the rear leg located on the inside of the thigh—about one-third of the way from the front of the leg.

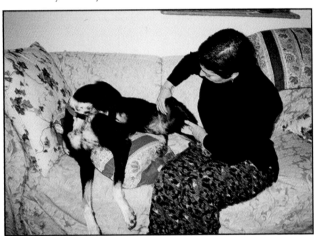

Applying Tourniquets

A tourniquet is any device that compresses a blood vessel to stop the bleeding of a tail or limb. As a last resort, apply a tourniquet for uncontrolled bleeding prior to and/or during transport to the hospital. The force exerted by a tourniquet is stronger than manual pressure alone. They should be used only when direct manual pressure and ice fail. Tourniquets can cause permanent injury if left on for longer than is absolutely necessary, although, in an emergency, the benefits far outweigh any risk.

If the wound is relatively small, place the tourniquet directly over a thick dressing. If the wound is large or there is no dressing, or if bleeding continues despite a tourniquet applied directly over the injured site, try placing the tourniquet 2 or 3 inches closer to the body. *Note:* In this position, and if the tourniquet successfully stops the flow of blood, a light dressing can be placed over the wound, but do not delay unnecessarily before seeking emergency treatment.

The simplest type of tourniquet can be made with bandaging material or a strip of cloth. Place a thick dressing of gauze squares, cloth or even a clean sanitary pad over the wound. Tie the tourniquet around the bleeding wound, or slightly above it if necessary, and tighten the knot until bleeding slows or stops completely.

Here is another way to fashion a tourniquet:

1. Tie a knot with the bandage or cloth strip over the injury or slightly above it.
2. Place a stick, spoon, pen or pencil over the first knot and tie a second knot around the object.
3. Tighten the knot and twist the stick-like object you have chosen until bleeding is controlled.
4. Lay the object parallel to the tail or limb and wrap in place with bandaging material.

Tourniquets are not comfortable for the victim (if he is conscious), but this is no time to worry about discomforting your dog. Your decision to apply a tourniquet was made because of uncontrolled hemorrhage. Transport *immediately.*

For a detailed discussion of how to dress a bleeding wound, and how to apply bandages and splints, see chapter 2.

Scratches and Punctures

SCRATCHES

A scratch (abrasion) can be caused by conflicts with other animals, but can also occur by contact with abrasive or jagged surfaces, such as rocks or certain plants. Superficial scratches generally require only light disinfection of the skin. For deep scratches, however, it is advisable to clip the hair to promote healing—apply an antibiotic ointment two to three times per day for at least seven days. Always watch for any signs of infection, such as redness, swelling, local heat, fever, pain or discharge (pus).

PUNCTURES

A puncture wound can be defined as any perforating injury that is deeper than it is wide. A puncture wound may be linear or circular. Puncture wounds may be the result of being bitten. A bite wound often has two puncture wounds that correspond to the upper canine

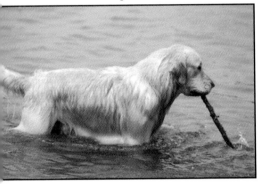

A puncture wound can result from a fall on a perforating object.

teeth of the aggressor, but there may be only one puncture wound caused by a bite if only one tooth made contact. Punctures may also be due to other causes, such as trauma from a knife or gunshot. A knife wound, for example, will cause a linear puncture (or stab wound). A bullet wound is generally circular at the point of entry and can be quite small depending on the bullet caliber. If there is an exit wound, it may be much larger and have irregular borders. Punctures can also result from a fall on a perforating object, such as a pointed stick, a pitchfork, a shard of broken glass or a metal fragment. If your dog has a puncture wound, there may be much bleeding or very little, depending on the location of the injury, the tissues that were damaged and the cause of injury. In the event of a puncture wound, you should:

- Evaluate the whole animal; is he agitated or is he unusually calm? Is the dog conscious or unresponsive? Can you find a heartbeat? Is the dog breathing?

- Look for signs of shock (see chapter 2), such as pale or pasty gums and a rapid pulse. Perform CPR as necessary; keep your pet warm; do not focus on disinfecting the wound or taking your dog's temperature.

- If there is profuse bleeding, apply direct pressure or a pressure bandage to the site; transport your dog to the nearest veterinary facility.

- If the wound penetrates the chest, a lung may have been punctured (hold your hand over the injury to feel for the passage of air that coincides with exhaling), major vessels may have been severed or the heart itself may have been lacerated. If necessary, press a clean or sterile dressing directly into the open wound to fill the space. Transport your dog to the nearest veterinary clinic *immediately.*

- If the perforating object has remained embedded in your dog, *do not remove the object!* The object itself may be controlling bleeding in deeper tissues by applying pressure against blood vessels. Moreover, by withdrawing the object you may cause additional damage and pain to your dog. Keep your dog warm and calm; transport him *immediately* to the nearest veterinary clinic (call ahead if you can so your dog can have immediate attention and treatment).

Whenever your dog is wounded, get as much information as possible about the circumstances surrounding the injury. The details could be important to help your veterinarian provide the appropriate treatments. For example, if the wound was caused by another animal, a rabies vaccine booster may be required, or if it was caused by a rusty nail, a tetanus antitoxin may be advisable.

Burns and Scalds

Burns can be caused by electrical cords or outlets, heat or fire, hot grease or oil, inhaled smoke and many corrosive chemicals. Scalds are caused by hot or boiling liquids, most typically hot water or spilled food items from the stove top or the oven. There are two major criteria used to evaluate the severity of these injuries:

1. The percentage of the body surface that was damaged, and
2. the depth of the burn.

- 1st degree—superficial: Pain, redness, blistering may occur; the hair may be singed but hair follicles remain firm; healing is usually uneventful and rapid;

- 2nd degree—moderate: Pain, redness, blistering are evident; the hair may remain firm; healing will be gradual;

- 3rd degree—severe: All layers of skin are destroyed, leaving a black or pearly white wound; the hair is destroyed; initially, there may be little or no pain; healing will leave serious scars unless plastic surgery is performed.

First degree burns that cover a small area (such as ½ square inch), usually require only basic first aid. If the sore starts to look moist, becomes very itchy or still looks red after two or three days, it should be seen by your veterinarian. Second or 3rd degree burns can be fatal if followed by shock, dehydration or infection. Depending on the severity of the injury, complications can be immediate or they can be delayed. Administer first aid and seek immediate veterinary attention.

First aid for very recent and minor 1st or 2nd degree burns or scalds:

1. Pour cool water over the burned area (use a garden hose, kitchen sink, cold shower) or apply an ice pack for at least twenty minutes.

2. Blot the area dry with a clean and dry cloth (do not use a material that will leave lint or other particles that could adhere to the sore area).

3. Clip the hair from the wound surface and a 1 inch margin around it using the tip of a blunt scissors or a clipper intended for use on pets.

4. Apply topical antibiotic ointment.

5. If your dog tries to lick the wound, place a sterile nonstick dressing and a light bandage to cover the area; change the dressing twice daily to keep the skin dry.

First aid for wide areas of 1st or 2nd degree burns or scalds and for any size 3rd degree burn:

1. Check for signs of shock (see chapter 2), keep your dog calm and cover him with a blanket if he is shivering.

2. If your dog shows no signs of shock (alert, completely normal behavior, gums pink, no difficulty breathing), apply a cool compress or ice pack to the injury for twenty minutes before seeking immediate veterinary care.

3. If your dog is showing signs of shock, seek veterinary care without delay.

First aid for chemical burns from an irritating or poisonous substance:

1. Protect your own skin with rubber or latex gloves (or any other glove that may be available) before you touch your dog; discard the gloves before touching anything else.

2. Remove and discard any collar, harness, bandanna or leash that could have been contaminated by the offending substance.

3. Wash your dog by repeatedly flushing with generous amounts of clear water (use a garden hose with a gentle stream of water or use your tub or shower).

4. Follow the water rinse with a bath using a liquid detergent (for hands or dish washing); work up a generous lather; rinse thoroughly and repeat.

5. Call your veterinarian's office for further instructions.

Your dog may burn or scald his mouth by licking a corrosive substance adhered to his coat (look for heavy

> **TO PREVENT BURNS AND SCALDS**
>
> Do not leave your dog unattended in a place with burning candles, lamps or any open flame, indoors or outdoors. Make sure that the screen to your fireplace is stable and that the door to your wood-burning stove is secure.
>
> Keep pot handles facing inward on the stove top or counter top and do not leave hot food items unguarded (especially on barbecues or grills) if your dog is prone to raiding for food. If you bathe your dog at home, use lukewarm (room temperature) water—test the water with your elbow before immersing him. Keep electrical cords covered, or off the ground so that they cannot be chewed. If cords cannot be rendered inaccessible, keep your dog out of that room.

drooling and unusual tongue movement), or by electrocution due to chewing on an electric cord or by simply investigating a hot object, such as a frying pan, with his mouth.

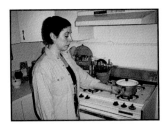

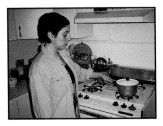

Turn pot handles inward on the stove to prevent access by your dog.

First aid for an oral burn: Rinse the dog's mouth liberally and repeatedly with clear water. Hold your garden hose for your dog to drink (*do not force the water down his throat*), give him an ice cube to chew on or use a gravy baster to flush cool water into his mouth. The oral cavity generally heals rapidly if you act quickly. If your dog has swallowed or licked a chemical compound, however, your next step should be to contact your veterinarian for further advice or to call the National Animal Poison Control Center at 1(800)548-2428. Some substances are highly toxic even in minute quantities and your dog may require additional emergency care by a trained professional.

Contact with Poison

Some poisons may be absorbed through the skin or mucous membranes. Poisons that may be ingested or inhaled are discussed in chapter 6. If your pet has been bitten by a snake or poisonous spider, apply an ice pack to the wound, keep your dog calm and take him to an emergency clinic right away. Try to describe the snake or spider in detail to help your veterinarian decide which treatment will be best. If your dog has come in contact (skin or hair) with an irritating or poisonous substance, protect your own skin with rubber or latex gloves (or any other glove that may be available) before you touch your dog. Remove any flea or tick collar that was placed on your dog's neck recently in case it is contributing to the problem. Wash your dog by repeatedly flushing with generous amounts of clear water (hose your dog down with a gentle stream of water in your yard, use your shower or fill the tub to his mid-chest level and ladle water with

a plastic or metal bowl or your hands, if necessary).
Follow this by bathing with a liquid detergent (for
hands or dish washing); work up a generous lather;
rinse thoroughly and repeat.

Allergic Reactions—Insect Bites and Stings

Allergy is a complex of extreme defensive reactions
directed against external or internal allergy-causing
substances or materials, collectively called allergens.

Allergic reactions are varied and can include itchiness,
hives, facial swelling, red and tearing eyes, sinus con-
gestion and sneezing, asthma, diarrhea and vomiting
and other internal responses that can even be fatal. In
clinical practice the treatment of allergy, for both people and other animals, involves:

- the identification of the allergen and its source,

- the prevention of contact with allergens,

- and the control of allergic symptoms with specific
  medication.

When allergens are unavoidable (for example, when
pollens fill the air beginning in the spring through the
first frost in the northeastern United States) then controlled desensitization by a series of injections offers
eventual relief to the allergy sufferer.

The control of mild to moderate allergic reaction is
accomplished by the administration of antihistamines,
which control the side effects of the allergic immune
response. Antihistamines may be prescribed by your
veterinarian to control your dog's allergy problems.
There are many different antihistamines and it is often
a trial and error process to find the one that works best
for your pet's symptoms. It should also be noted that
an antihistamine may work well for a while and then
lose its effectiveness, making it necessary to prescribe
another one instead. In cases where the allergic response has progressed to more considerable discomfort, other medications may be necessary.

Insects such as bees, wasps, hornets, flies, ants, ticks, fleas, spiders and mosquitoes can all leave their mark on your dog. Luckily, only a few will produce urgent situations. Most insect bites simply result in localized pain or itchiness. Removal of the insects with tweezers (if a tick) or pesticides (if your dog has fleas), and short-term management of related symptoms with an antihistamine or a corticosteroid are usually all that is required to resolve the problem.

Some spider bites, such as that of the black widow spider, trigger more than just a local allergic reaction. The black widow delivers a poisonous bite that initially will cause local pain and swelling before progressing to generalized body pain, weakness and fever.

Your puppy (and child) are susceptible to insect bites when outdoors, but only some will produce urgent situations.

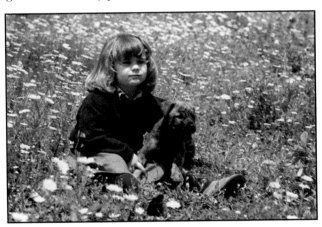

Bee stings are painful but a dog that is predisposed to bee sting allergy could develop serious complications to a second bee sting. The first time the dog is stung he may experience some local swelling, or the reaction may be so mild that it may go unnoticed. If the dog is stung in the face, a common occurrence, then some facial swelling may be obvious. Facial swelling can progress to involve the upper airways and throat, however, and could obstruct the passage of air to the lungs. Facial swelling is serious and warrants prompt first aid.

If you discover a swollen and itchy area on your dog's skin, part the hair to see if you can detect a biting insect, any obvious redness or the presence of a stinger embedded in the skin. A bee stinger, for example, looks like a very small (approximately 1/8 inch) fish-hook and is easily removed with tweezers. Administer 50 mg Benadryl (or its generic equivalent, Diphenhydramine) in tablet, capsule or liquid form. Keep this over-the-counter medication on hand in your medicine cabinet and/or in your dog's first aid kit. Apply an ice pack to the area to help control the itchiness and to minimize swelling. Call your veterinary clinic to report the incident, your dog's symptoms and current condition, and to ask for further recommendations.

If you discover that your dog has a swollen muzzle and puffy eyes, hives (skin swellings that resemble coins or bumps) that are spreading over the dog's body and/or severe itchiness anywhere on the body, you should *immediately* administer 50 mg of Benadryl (or its generic equivalent, Diphenhydramine). It may take as long as half an hour for the drug to begin its effect and allergy-related symptoms may take up to half a day to subside. Even if your dog seems to feel more comfortable shortly after antihistamine administration, schedule a veterinary visit within twenty-four hours to prevent any

Use tweezers to remove ticks from your dog.

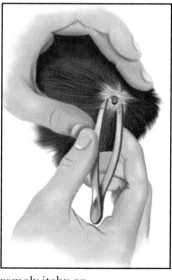

relapse and to plan on what to do if there is another episode. When facial swelling is present, however, call your veterinarian right away and have your dog seen *immediately*, even if he seems unbothered by his swollen face (which is unlikely).

Itchy Dog

A very itchy dog can lose sleep and weight, prevent his owner from sleeping, vocalize excessively, chew and scratch obsessively and even self-mutilate. Itchiness can come on gradually over many days or weeks or it can "explode" with little warning in its most intense form. If your dog is extremely itchy or uncomfortable, and could cause himself injury, then an itch is definitely an urgent symptom.

If your dog appears to be itchy, part his hair and investigate.

- Look for a tick—remove the tick with a tweezers by firmly grasping its head as close to the dog's skin as possible. (Kill the insect by soaking it in alcohol or nail polish remover, or hold it up to a small flame so that it is dead before you discard it.)

- If you see a flea or black specks on the skin (these are flea feces and will stain reddish brown in a drop of water), treat your pet for flea infestation. Call your veterinary clinic for advice on current advances in flea and tick control.

- The skin may be red or blotchy, or you may find an infected sore, a puncture wound or a scratch. Clip the hair carefully with the tip of a blunt scissors and disinfect the area. Make an appointment for your dog to be seen at the first available opening.

- If you do not see any obvious explanation for your dog's discomfort, schedule a veterinary visit as soon as possible; bring a stool (fecal) sample with you in case it is called for; additional laboratory tests may be advised.

- Note the area(s) where your dog is itchy, whether the discomfort has worsened since you first noticed it and exactly how long he has been uncomfortable so that you can relay important details to your veterinarian.

If your dog is more than just a little itchy, administer the antihistamine Benadryl (or its generic equivalent, Diphenhydramine) by mouth. Twenty-five mg is an appropriate dose for small dogs (under 30 pounds); give 50mg to medium- or large-sized dogs. You may repeat this every eight hours, if necessary, until your veterinary visit; be sure to tell your veterinarian that you gave this medication to your dog and at which dose. When antihistamine alone does not ease your dog's distress you may apply an ice pack to the itchy spot(s) for at least five minutes.

For extreme itchiness, or if the itchiness is over a wide area or even generalized to the entire body, it may be necessary to prevent your dog from self-mutilation. An Elizabethan collar ("E collar," named for the fashionable wide collars worn in Elizabethan England) is intended

to keep your dog from licking or chewing himself from the neck downward and from scratching or rubbing at his head. The height of the collar must be at least 1 or 2 inches longer than your dog's nose. You can fabricate an E collar by cutting a hole in a plastic bucket or flower pot and tying it to your dog's collar with string. You can also make one by cutting a hole in the bottom of a cardboard box, or use a wide strip of cardboard or plastic to fashion a cone-shaped collar around your

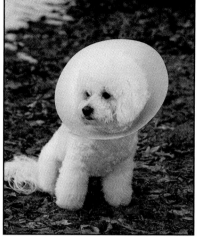

dog's head. Alternatively, your veterinary clinic can supply a ready-made E collar until your scheduled appointment. Think of the E collar as damage control until your veterinarian can examine your dog and relieve any discomfort.

An Elizabethan collar will keep your dog from licking or chewing himself from the neck down.

Paw Problems

A dog's foot is subject to a lot of abuse on a daily basis. *Get your dog accustomed to having his feet and toes touched* by gently manipulating these areas daily. Start when your dog is young—before an urgent problem develops. You may want to give your dog a small food treat to reward his tolerance of your probing between his toes, applying gentle pressure to his foot pads and feet and lifting each foot for examination. In case you need to examine the feet in an emergency or simply to trim his toe nails, what an advantage you will have if your dog has been trained to tolerate this in advance!

If your dog has cut his paw, chances are there will be quite a bit of bleeding. The foot pads are thick but once the surface is lacerated, highly vascularized (with a high concentration of blood vessels) tissue is exposed to injury. Apply direct pressure, or better yet, direct pressure with an ice pack. If bleeding continues or the cut appears deep, call your veterinarian to let him or her know that your dog needs immediate attention. Continue direct pressure on the drive down or apply a pressure bandage. Do not panic—this is not a fatal injury, just a messy one!

If the cut seems superficial and bleeding is absent or easily controlled, flush the wound with lukewarm water. Follow with a five-minute foot soak in a small basin or bowl containing about ½ inch of water (enough to cover the injury) mixed with a capful of bleach. *Note:* The feet are very contaminated and easily become infected; bleach is a wonderful disinfectant and, although it may sting elsewhere on the body, its use is appropriate for the feet. Rinse again with clear water and pat the foot dry. Apply an antibiotic ointment, a dressing and a bandage. Change the bandage and dressing daily: Repeat the foot soak, flush with clear water and pat dry; reapply the ointment before the clean dressing is applied.

You should arrange for a prompt veterinary visit if: the cut produces a discharge resembling pus, fails to close, the borders and surrounding area become red, there is a lack of improvement after three to five days or pain or fever are present.

Swollen paws or toes may be caused by fractured bones, blunt trauma, soft tissue injury (such as torsion or sprains), infections, foreign bodies, insect bites, bandages that are too tightly applied or elastic bands that obstruct circulation. If your dog seems to be limping or licking at his feet:

1. Remove any bandage or dressing that may be too tight because it was applied before swelling was noticed, and call your veterinarian to reapply the bandage. If you applied the bandage

---

AVOID INJURIES BY TRAVELING SAFELY

To keep your dog safe while in a car, place him in a travel cage or crate that will not shift in the vehicle. Safety belts for dogs are another option.

Do *not* let your dog ride with his head out of the window, regardless of how much he may enjoy it. This practice leads to eye injuries and even ejection from the car should you have an accident. Similarly, do *not* let your dog ride in the back of a pick-up truck—he can be easily jostled and hurt or thrown from the vehicle altogether.

yourself, make an appointment for the vet to examine the paw.

2. Closely examine the dog's feet:

- Hold the paw, without squeezing or twisting it, and gently separate the toes to examine between them; do the same under the foot and examine each foot pad; look for any crack or cut on the foot pads or the skin between them; watch for broken, bleeding or infected toenails.

- Make sure there is no red, moist or swollen area, or any unusual odor.

- Use your fingers to double check for the presence of any penetrating splinter or foreign object, such as a sticky burr or insect stinger, which may be very small; remove what you find with tweezers.

3. If your dog's foot is causing him great pain, or if you can see or feel "crunching in the foot," there may be fractured bones. Apply an ice pack, if possible, to minimize swelling and pain—bring your pet to the veterinarian the same day.

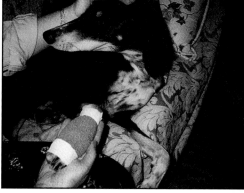

4. If you do not suspect a fracture and find only a small area of irritation (or nothing obvious at all), soak the foot in a basin or bowl of soapy, lukewarm water, running your fingers between each toe and foot pad, and rinse thoroughly in clear water before patting dry. This will disinfect the foot and, hopefully, remove any tiny splinters or insect barbs that remain undetected; also, any irritating substance on the skin or hair surface should be washed away.

To bandage a dog's paw, apply the bandage and tape over the gauze dressing and layers of rolled gauze.

5. If a toenail is broken or bleeding, flush debris by soaking in clear water and wrap the nail in a

nonstick dressing and bandage and have your dog seen within twenty-four hours.

6. If there is no obvious reason for the licking or lameness, work your way up the dog's leg to search for any swelling or wound between the foot and the shoulder. If your dog seems otherwise unaffected (playful, eating well), schedule a veterinary appointment within twenty-four to forty-eight hours.

7. Regardless of whether you detect a problem, if your pet stops eating or is in real discomfort, see your veterinarian as soon as possible.

Sometimes sticky substances (like bubble gum, tree sap or tar) can adhere to the hair on a dog's feet (or anywhere else) or to foot pads. Carefully snip the soiled hairs away with the tip of a blunt scissors. Alternatively, hold an ice cube against the sticky stuff to make it harden—it will be easier to peel away.

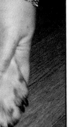

INGROWN TOENAILS

A dog's toenails can grow long and curve downward to penetrate the foot pads. This is called an ingrown toenail. Dogs that enjoy healthy amounts of exercise generally wear down the toenails on asphalt or pavement. Nonetheless, trimming your dog's nails is part of a good grooming habit, and will greatly diminish the likelihood of the formation of ingrown nails.

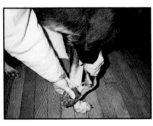

Examine the foot between the toes from the top as well as the pads of the feet. Do not twist the foot or leg during your inspection.

A dog with arthritis in his feet may have twisted or deformed toes that do not place the toenail in an optimum position for wear. In addition, the dew claws, located about one-fourth of the way up on the inside of the leg, have no contact with the ground and may curl around and become embedded in the leg. Toenails that have become ingrown are painful and have a high incidence of infection.

- Trim the nail and pry it gently from the puncture wound it has created.

- Disinfect with hydrogen peroxide (for foot injuries, diluted bleach is an acceptable alternative) on a cotton ball or gauze.

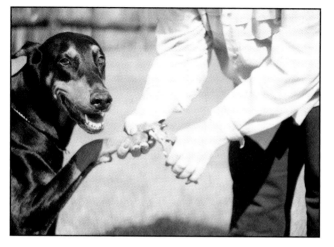

Reduce the incidence of ingrown toenails with regular nail trimming.

- Apply a topical antibiotic.

- To keep the sore clean until it heals closed, repeat the above process when the dog returns from an outing.

- It is usually unnecessary to apply a bandage unless the sore is open, but if your dog is licking at the site, cover it with a light dressing for two or three days; clean with disinfectant, reapply antibiotic ointment and replace the dressing daily.

- If there continues to be any pus, foul smelling discharge, swelling, fever or discomfort after several days, see your veterinarian as soon as possible.

Internal Problems

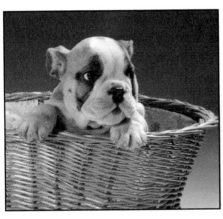

Bloat

Gastric dilatation and torsion, more commonly referred to as "bloat," occurs when the stomach bloats with gases and twists around itself. The result is one of the most serious emergencies that dog owners and veterinarians can encounter. The symptoms for bloat follow a rapid sequence—

- the abdomen expands as the stomach bloats,

- the dog may show signs of abdominal discomfort (looks at her sides, seems restless, anxious),

- difficulty breathing develops (rapid and shallow) as the bloated abdomen compresses against the diaphragm and major vessels,

- the color of the tongue may take on a pale or whitish tinge,

- the dog collapses on her side as vascular compression and the release of toxins into the bloodstream progresses,

- death results from cardiac arrest or shock.

These events may occur over several hours or within a single hour, depending on how rapidly the stomach bloats and/or twists. For some lucky dogs, the stomach will bloat but not rotate. Gastric distention is still an emergency, but the prognosis is better than bloat with rotation (dilatation and torsion).

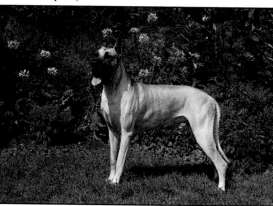

Certain dog breeds, such as Great Danes and St. Bernards and mixed breeds with certain body types, are more prone to gastric bloat. Bloat can occur at any age and may affect the same dog more than once in her lifetime. Emergency surgery is the only treatment. Both surgery and the postoperative recuperation period can be complicated.

Some breeds, like the Great Dane, are more prone than others to developing gastric bloat.

First aid for gastric bloating is limited:

1. If your dog's abdomen is obviously swollen (looks and feels like a balloon begin inflated) and she is showing signs consistent with those described above: Find a medium-sized safety pin or sewing needle (pour alcohol over it or pass it through a small flame if you have time to sterilize it). With your fingers, trace the end of the rib cage and find the area of either side of the abdomen that feels the most like a balloon. With a rapid jab, pass the needle into the dog's side just as you would pop a balloon—the purpose of this is to allow some of the gases to escape so that the gastric distention

can be reduced, at least temporarily. See a veterinarian *immediately!*

2. If your dog's belly is only slightly expanded, but she otherwise seems relatively comfortable *OR* if the belly is showing no distention but the dog is showing unusual signs of abdominal discomfort: Do not attempt first aid; call the clinic to let them know you are coming in with your dog right away.

Bowel Disorders

DIARRHEA

Diarrhea *may* present an urgent situation, but a bout of diarrhea is not automatically an emergency. Diarrhea is common in dogs and functions primarily to rid the digestive system of noxious contents.

**HELP TO
PREVENT BLOAT**

If your dog has a history of gastric distention and/or torsion or fits the body type of predisposed breeds, you may decrease the chance of her suffering from bloat. Feed your dog several small meals a day instead of one or two larger meals. Avoid highly energetic exercise within an hour or two after mealtime. Prevent your dog from drinking excessively immediately after feeding (give her a cup of water every hour rather than leaving a full bowl accessible). Soak dry food with lukewarm water before serving your dog's meal.

Diarrhea becomes a serious consideration if it is associated with fever, decreased appetite, vomiting or increasing lethargy. It is also a serious condition when the stools become very liquid, contain more than a drop of blood or if it continues for more than one or two days. If you have any concern, call the clinic to have your dog examined. Bring a fecal sample, so that the veterinarian can check for the presence of internal parasites. Diarrhea can result in dehydration, electrolyte imbalance and, in extreme cases, shock.

In puppies younger than 6 months of age, diarrhea can result in rapid decline. The younger the pup, the more critical it is to obtain quick veterinary intervention. Do not wait to call for professional advice—your puppy should be seen on the same day as the diarrhea appears.

Adult dogs in poor health or dogs over 10 years old should also be examined as soon as possible.

If there is more than just a drop or two of blood or if the diarrhea (pasty or liquid stools) is the color of dark chocolate or darker, call for an immediate veterinary visit.

If the diarrhea has not subsided (e.g., less frequent elimination, stools become firmer, dog seems more comfortable) within twenty-four hours of implementing the recommendations that follow below, your pet should be seen by a veterinarian right away.

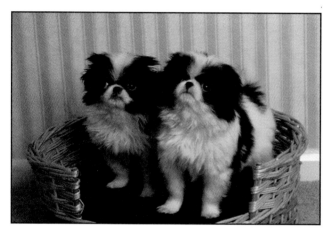

In young puppies, diarrhea can be a serious condition—your puppy should be taken to the veterinarian right away.

If your dog develops diarrhea but is otherwise un-affected:

- Place her on a bland diet consisting of boiled chicken or hamburger meat mixed with boiled or steamed rice.

- Feed smaller, more frequent meals (three or four per day) of this special mix until stools solidify and become normal.

- When bowel movements are firm, mix your dog's regular food with the bland diet for two or three days before discontinuing the rice mixture.

- If you have any lingering concern, call your veterinarian to report the problem and your dog's current status in case your pet should still be seen. Ask the veterinarian if he or she would like you to bring in a fecal sample.

71

If your dog develops diarrhea and seems slightly sluggish or if she is also vomiting:

- Follow the plan outlined above, but also try the following additional suggestions.

- Measure your dog's rectal temperature (see chapter 2); if it is elevated (higher than 103°), call the clinic for further advice.

- If the dog's temperature is normal, remove food and water (including treats) for twenty-four hours. If she has not vomited in the last eight hours, you may give her an ice cube to lick every few hours for the remainder of the fasting period, as long as she does not vomit. Reintroduce food by feeding a bland diet in small and frequent meals as described above.

- If vomiting or diarrhea resume when food is reintroduced, remove food and water; call your veterinarian for further advice.

KEEP YOUR DOG FIT TO HELP PREVENT DISEASE

A healthy, balanced diet with limited (or no) "snacking" will go far to keep your dog fit. Obesity is a serious problem for dogs—they are more likely to become ill if they are overweight, and they are more difficult to medically treat. Similarly, regular exercise is important to maintaining good muscle tone and cardiac fitness. A daily routine of walking and playing will also keep your dog from becoming bored—and will make her less likely to be destructive in the home.

CONSTIPATION

Constipation can be extremely uncomfortable for your dog. The absence of stools can be expected following a bout of diarrhea, for example, when bowel movements may be absent for a day or two. If the dog is eating and behaving normally, production should soon resume. Constipation is not an urgent symptom but should be considered serious if your pet has kidney disease, diabetes or any physical condition that predisposes her to dehydration. Also, if your dog is chronically constipated due to rectal dysfunction you will need to monitor stool production more closely. If apparent constipation is accompanied by vomiting or any sign of abdominal distress, have your dog examined by a veterinarian right away to be sure there is no intestinal obstruction. If you see a piece of string, thread or ribbon protruding from the anus *do not pull it out!* This could lacerate the intestines and create a real emergency. Carefully trim the protruding filament to about ½ inch from the anus and, as long as your dog behaves normally, follow the home remedy for constipation below:

- If stools are not produced for more than forty-eight hours, you may add 2 teaspoons, 2 tablespoons or up to ¼ cup (depending on the size of your dog) of bran cereal to your dog's meals; alternatively, mix one-half of the adult dose of psyllium or Metamucil in her food.

- Encourage water intake as well as daily exercise. If bowel function does not resume normally within forty-eight hours, your dog should be examined and the choice of any additional treatment should be left to professionals. *Do not administer laxatives or enemas to your dog without specific veterinary instruction.*

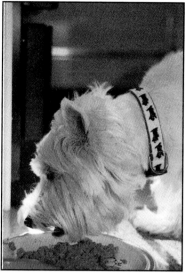

If your dog becomes constipated, try mixing a little bran cereal or psyllium into her food.

Diabetic Emergencies

Insulin is a pancreatic hormone that is required in the metabolism of glucose, the major fuel used by the body's cells. Diabetes is a complex disease caused by an insufficient natural supply of insulin and requires cooperation between you and your veterinarian.

Without insulin, or when a confirmed diabetic fails to respond to insulin injection at the recommended dose, the glucose level rises in the blood stream and the resulting symptoms are associated with the body's attempts to adjust. Excessive thirst and excessive urination occur as the diabetic's body tries to dilute the concentration of glucose. Eventually, compensating mechanisms fail and deterioration, once begun, can be rapid.

73

When diabetes is diagnosed, insulin replacement therapy (by subcutaneous injection once or twice daily) is begun. With too high an insulin dose, the blood glucose level may plummet. With its vital fuel supply devastated, the body collapses. The brain is the most sensitive organ to low blood glucose and thus tremors, seizure and the diabetic coma ensue.

If your dog drinks more than usual, urinates excessively, has a strange sweet smell to her breath, seems more subdued than usual and is losing weight, she may be an unconfirmed or uncontrolled diabetic. Schedule an appointment with your veterinarian to investigate further.

If your dog is diabetic, carefully follow your veterinarian's directions on how to fill the prescribed

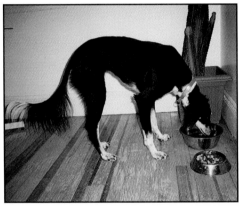

amount of insulin into the syringe and how to administer a subcutaneous injection (described in chapter 2). The most common reason that dogs fail to respond to insulin injection is improper technique in administering the medication.

If your dog is a confirmed diabetic and is being regu-

Excessive thirst is a common sign of high blood pressure associated with uncontrolled diabetes.

lated with insulin injections, keep corn syrup or some other form of liquid glucose on hand in case her blood sugar drops. Because the body's metabolism is a dynamic process, blood sugar may drop even if the correct dose of insulin is administered.

Blood glucose will be at its lowest level approximately four to eight hours after insulin administration, although it may begin to drop sooner. To prevent glucose levels from plunging too rapidly, give your dog a small meal about four to eight hours after insulin. If your dog seems uncoordinated, confused, is shaking or very sleepy four to eight hours after her insulin injection, her glucose levels may have dropped too low. Give her about 1 teaspoon of sweet syrup directly into her mouth, repeating every fifteen minutes or so until she seems more alert and responsive. Feed her a small meal of her regular food and call your veterinarian right away for further advice. If your dog, about four to eight hours after insulin, is dazed and unresponsive, or loses consciousness and cannot be aroused , rub 1 teaspoon of syrup directly onto her gums; cover her with a blanket and take her to the veterinarian *immediately.*

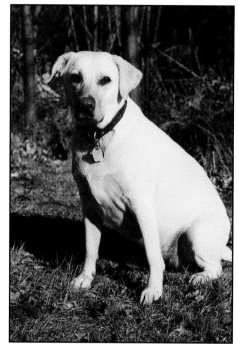

If your dog goes into convulsions four to eight hours after insulin administration, very carefully lift her upper lip and drizzle the teaspoon of syrup onto her gums and release. Do not risk being bitten—your dog is unconscious during a seizure and cannot control her jaws. Cover her with a blanket and see your veterinarian *immediately.*

A diabetic dog that is vomiting, has diarrhea or has a fever should be seen by a veterinarian within twenty-four hours. In the interim, call the clinic for advice on how to adjust the insulin dose before your scheduled appointment.

Obesity in dogs makes it more difficult to control diabetes.

If you are late or miss giving your dog her scheduled injection, administer the recommended insulin dose and call the clinic for further directions.

Drug Sensitivities

Your dog may have a negative response to a medication prescribed to treat an unrelated illness. If she is on a course of medication and seems increasingly lethargic or unusually calm, stops eating, develops vomiting or diarrhea or starts to scratch, bite or rub herself, she may be showing signs of drug intolerance or sensitivity. Adverse drug reactions can develop with any medication, even with aspirin, and suspected problems should be reported to your veterinarian without delay.

If you suspect that your dog is negatively affected by any medication or medicinal preparation, contact your veterinarian without delay. *It is usually better not to discontinue a prescription without your veterinarian's instruction to do so.* Your veterinarian should be given the opportunity to determine whether the treatment is the cause of the problem or whether the underlying medical problem is failing to respond to the prescribed treatment. Call to make an appointment right away. Do not dismiss any concern you have regarding your dog's health.

Note: Make certain that any suspected drug sensitivities are noted prominently on your dog's medical record. You should also keep a record of the drug name and the symptoms that developed from its use in case your dog is treated elsewhere and her file is unavailable for reference.

DIABETES AND WEIGHT CONTROL

By maintaining your dog's ideal body weight, you will maximize her response to treatment. If she is obese, get advice on how to gradually reduce her weight to prevent diseases associated with obesity, such as diabetes. Add 1 teaspoon or tablespoon of bran cereal (depending on the size of your dog) to her food to help absorb some of the excess glucose in the intestine before it is absorbed. This should help to regulate your dog's glucose level, the amount of insulin needed and, as an added bonus, the regularity of bowel habits!

Urinary Problems

Urinary tract problems are diverse, and include obstruction, infection, incontinence, inflammation, malformation and traumatic injuries, among many others. Sudden onset of kidney failure or complete urinary obstruction, for example, can have fatal consequences if left untreated. Fortunately, most urinary tract diseases are not immediately life-threatening, although they can cause discomfort. Bladder infections, for example, can become extremely painful to the dog. Dieases of the male dog's prostate gland can cause symptoms that must be distinguished from bladder infections, and the prostate should be routinely examined in both neutered and intact males. Other problems, such as urinary incontinence, are more distressing to the owner than to the dog. Remember, however, that an emergency should be defined partly by your dog's level of comfort and your level of concern. Symptoms associated with urinary tract problems include—

- increased frequency of urination,
- increased volume of urination,
- pain during urination,
- pink, brownish or reddish color of urine,
- straining to urinate,
- inability to pass urine,
- increased frequency of drinking,
- increase volume of water intake,
- licking at penis or vulva (with or without discharge),
- inappropriate urination inside your home.

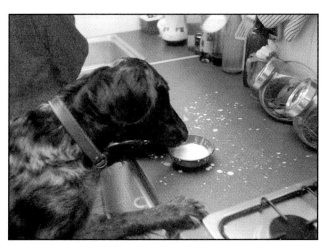

Increased frequency of drinking is a sign of a urinary tract infection.

Many of these same symptoms are common to several urinary ailments or are associated with problems that are unrelated to the urinary system. However, if any of these signs develop in your dog, she deserves veterinary attention within twenty-four hours. If your dog is straining to urinate, seems unable to urinate or has pain, see a veterinarian on the same day. If, in addition to any of these symptoms, your dog also has a fever, stops eating or drinking and becomes sluggish or withdrawn, see a veterinarian *immediately*. Whenever possible, try to collect a fresh urine specimen and, unless you leave within an hour or two, refrigerate it until you are on your way to the clinic. However, do not delay transport in an emergency in order to obtain a urine sample.

Uterine and Vaginal Problems

The average female dog reaches sexual maturity at about 6 months of age. In large breeds this may be delayed to the age of 10 months or older. Estrus ("heat") normally occurs every six months and usually lasts about one to three weeks. Your female pup will not benefit, either behaviorally or physically, by coming into estrus even once, nor does she require the experience of producing a litter to lead a happy life. In fact, the opposite may be true—young pups may have a vaginal discharge that ranges from cloudy white to shades of yellow. This is most often caused by vaginal infections that are very difficult to treat. Should this occur, make a veterinary appointment at your earliest convenience. Antibiotics may be helpful temporarily, but spay surgery by the age of 6 months is curative.

Vaginal discharge (mucus, pus of any color) in dogs of any age should receive veterinary attention as soon as possible. Vaginal discharge is normal for several weeks following delivery of puppies and may range in color from brownish-red to dark chocolate brown to greenish-brown—as long as the bitch is behaving normally and the puppies are healthy this should not be of concern.

DO NOT INTERFERE WITH MATING DOGS

During mating, the male's penis becomes engorged with blood and remains locked in the female's vagina for up to about thirty minutes until erection recedes. Following ejaculation, the male may turn around until he is tail to tail with the female but remains locked in place. Do not try to separate them! This could cause serious and unnecessary injury to both dogs—let nature take its course and deal with the consequences once the pair separate of their own accord.

Bloody vaginal discharge is common during estrus—the vulva will be swollen, the bitch will seem restless, will urinate in small amounts and more often and may be irritable. *Do not leave her unattended anywhere outside your home!*

Bloody vaginal discharge in a spayed female or a female that is not in heat should receive prompt, immediate veterinary attention. The urgency of the condition is directly proportional to the abundance of the bleeding. Vaginal bleeding in any dog that is accompanied by discomfort, fever, loss of appetite, lethargy or agitation should also prompt an emergency visit right away.

Vaginal discharge, discomfort, fever, loss of appetite, lethargy or restlessness in a bitch several days after mating could be signs of infection or laceration. If your dog has these symptoms, call for an immediate appointment.

VAGINAL OR UTERINE PROLAPSE

The vagina and/or uterus may turn inside out and protrude to the outside of the body. Vaginal or uterine prolapse is an emergency situation that requires urgent veterinary intervention and surgery may be necessary. Left untreated, these conditions may become complicated by infection and obstructed blood supply. If your dog is distressed and licking at what looks like a red gelatinous cauliflower of any size (it may be quite large if the prolapse is uterine) protruding from the vulva, you should:

1. Flush with cold water gently poured over the pulpy mass. Wear latex or rubber gloves if these are

SPAY YOUR FEMALE DOG

To prevent common emergencies in your bitch, have her spayed! You will dramatically decrease her risk of malignant mammary tumors (the equivalent of breast cancer in women) and eliminate complications of pregnancy and delivery, false pregnancy, uterine and vaginal infections, ovarian disease, unintended breeding and the addition of puppies to the tragic proportions of the pet over-population crisis.

After spay surgery, follow your veterinarian's advice carefully. Keep your pet under controlled exercise until you are told to return her activity to normal. Watch for any type of discharge vaginally or from the incision site. If any sign of pain or discomfort is shown, call your veterinarian for further advice.

Complications following any surgery do occur, but serious complications are infrequent and should not discourage you from spaying your dog.

available, otherwise you will need to use bare hands that are thoroughly washed.

2. Sprinkle salt generously over the surface of the prolapse. After several minutes you should see the tissue begin to shrink; try to push the prolapse back into the vagina with several closed fingers (to avoid perforating the fragile tissues with just one finger).

3. If necessary, flush with cool water, apply salt and try to invert the prolapse once or twice more.

4. Regardless of whether you are successful, take your dog to a nearby veterinary facility right away. Cover the area with a clean damp towel to keep prolapsed tissues moist and to minimize contamination and trauma—even if you successfully reduced the prolapse, tissues can evert easily at any time, so a damp towel will be a good thing to take along.

5. If the exposed tissue has any areas that are brown, black or green, or if you detect any tears or puncture wounds on the surface, be sure to inform the veterinary staff. In these cases, spay surgery may be unavoidable to save your dog.

Pregnancy may be undesirable in the bitch for a number of reasons. She may be in poor physical health, or too old to withstand giving birth. She may also be too young—a bitch under 2 years of age is at a higher risk for complications at delivery. She may have been bred to a male that is too large, for example, a Beagle bitch should not be bred to a Newfoundland male. If a mismating has occurred and you would like to prevent fertilization, the following recommendations are offered:

FALSE PREGNANCY

False pregnancy is the display of physical and behavioral signs consistent with pregnancy in intact (not spayed), nonpregnant bitches. The vulva may be swollen, the belly may become enlarged and the mammary glands may even produce milk. The bitch may prepare a nest and carry toys or other objects to the spot. She may be restless, irritable and even aggressive. This is not an emergency and often resolves without treatment. Recurrence is common in subsequent estral cycles, however, and unless the dog is of particular breeding value she should be spayed to prevent this and all other vaginal or uterine disease.

---

1. See your veterinarian within forty-eight hours of mismating. Medication, by injection or by mouth,

is available to prevent pregnancy. It will also pro-
long the signs of "heat" by at least one week and
you will need to supervise her continually until
all signs of heat disappear. This
treatment will not prevent additional mismating!

. As mentioned elsewhere in this
book, get your dog spayed!

Poison Ingestion

Poisons can be found in common
household items, such as bleach or
house plants, or in automotive supplies, such as antifreeze or motor
oil. Pesticides and rodenticides are
poisonous, as are many paints and
shellac. Turpentine, kerosene, ace-
tone (found in nail polish remover)
and most cleaning fluids are dangerous to dogs, as are medicines
intended for human use, and illi-
cit drugs. Other potentially toxic
items include children's crayons
and shoe polish. Some food items,
such as chocolate, can be lethal. Finally, some poisons are found in
the environment, and may be contaminants (such as lawn and garden
herbicides or gasoline-polluted
water) or naturally occurring (such
as certain mushrooms or blue-green
algae).

The specific treatment for poisoning will depend on the poison in
question. Some poisons require
specific treatments and antidotes
whereas others call for basic life
support until the dog can clear the poison from her
system. There are, however, general first aid steps that
you can take immediately upon discovering that your
dog has ingested a poisonous substance:

Internal
Problems

TAKE STEPS TO PREVENT POISONING

Pet-proof your home as soon as
you acquire a dog and maintain
her safety for a lifetime! Make a
search of each room in your
home. Place toxic chemicals out of
reach or locked away safely. Place
safety latches (intended for child-
proofing) on all low cabinets that
are at the same level as your dog
and place gates to barricade your
dog from areas of your home that
might contain hazards. Minimize
your use of poisonous substances
altogether. Ask your mechanic to
substitute regular antifreeze with
the new generation of pet safe
antifreeze. Remove dangerous
plants from your home and your
yard. A partial listing of dangerous plants is provided in this chapter. Keep the telephone numbers of
your regular veterinary clinic and
local veterinary emergency center
in plain view (on your refrigerator,
for example) and on an index card
in your dog's first aid kit. Include
the hotline number of the National
Animal Poison Control Center—
1(800)548-2428 or 1 (888) 4ANI-
HELP. This organization, available
twenty-four hours a day, every
day, all year, is affiliated with the
ASPCA (American Society for the
Prevention of Cruelty to Animals).
The charge for the call is about
$30, but it will certainly be worth-
while in an emergency.

81

1. Induce vomiting by pouring a teaspoonful of either hydrogen peroxide or table salt on the dog's tongue as close to the back of the throat as possible.

   Note: If your dog has swallowed a corrosive chemical, such as a solvent or cleaning fluid, *do not induce vomiting.*

2. Collect a sample of your dog's vomit for laboratory analysis to identify an unknown poison.

3. Call ahead and proceed calmly to your veterinarian.

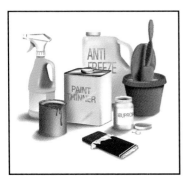

Some of the many household substances harmful to your dog.

If your dog has licked some of the substance adhered to her coat (look for heavy salivating and a licking motion with her tongue), rinse her mouth liberally with repeated clear water flushes and call your veterinarian's office for further instructions.

If your pet seems to be behaving normally after contact with poison, call your veterinarian for further emergency instructions or contact the National Animal Poison Control Center at 1(800)548-2428. Assuming that your veterinarian will want to see your dog, bring the prescription bottle of ingested medication, the package label of the ingested poison or a sample of the suspected source of poisoning so that your veterinarian can administer the specific treatment whenever possible.

If your pet seems to be deteriorating despite first aid, call your veterinary clinic to advise them that you will be arriving shortly and transport your pet *immediately* (along with anything that might identify the specific poison involved).

Vomiting

Vomiting is common in dogs and frequently serves to rid the body of harmful substances.

Vomiting can occur soon after swallowing an offending substance, or it can be delayed by many hours. It is a nonspecific response to dozens of physical and emotional causes that frequently must be excluded, one by one, with laboratory testing and careful physical examination. Assist your veterinarian in making a diagnosis by reporting details, which include: How long after a meal your dog vomited, how many times she has vomited in the last twenty-four hours, how many days the vomiting has continued and the appearance and contents of the vomited matter.

Vomiting takes on more serious implications in very young pups, dogs older than 10 years of age and adult dogs in poor health. Contact your veterinarian *immediately* if vomiting occurs in young, old or sick dogs. For example, diabetic dogs may need to decrease their daily insulin requirements or may need to be examined. Excessive vomiting can result in dehydration, electrolyte imbalance and, in extreme cases, shock. Seek professional advice within twenty-four hours if vomiting persists despite the suggestions that follow:

1. Measure your dog's rectal temperature (see chapter 2). If it is higher than 103°F, call the clinic for an appointment the same day.

2. If the dog's temperature is within normal range, remove food and water (including treats) for twenty-four hours. If your dog has not vomited in the last eight hours, you may give her an ice cube to lick every few hours for the remainder of the fasting period, as long as she

---

POISONOUS PLANTS

Poisonous ornamental plants: Note that this list is not all-inclusive.

Amaryllis

Azalea

Black-eyed Susan

Bleeding heart

Cone flower

Chinaberry tree

Daffodil

Euonymus

Foxglove

Hemlock

Horse chestnut

Hyacinth

Hydrangea

Iris

Larkspur

Lily-of-the-valley

Mistletoe

Oleander

Poinsettia

Poppy

Rhododendron

Snow-on-the-mountain

Star-of-Bethlehem

Virginia creeper

Wisteria

Yew

does not vomit. Do not be tempted to feed or water your dog before the twenty-four hours are over, even if she seems hungry and behaves normally, because you may precipitate more vomiting.

3. After twenty-four hours, place your dog on a bland diet consisting of boiled chicken or hamburger meat mixed with boiled or steamed rice. Feed smaller and more frequent meals (three or four per day) of this special mix for two to three days before gradually reintroducing her regular food.

Contact your veterinarian right away if your puppy is vomiting.

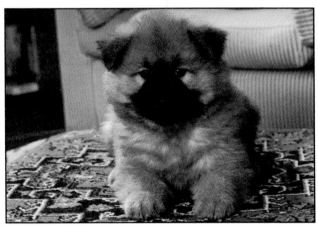

4. If vomiting resumes when food is reintroduced, remove food and water; call your veterinarian for further advice.

Heart Failure

Cardiac problems are relatively common in dogs and obesity plays a significant role in the development and progression of heart disease. With regular exercise and a controlled diet, dogs can maintain a healthy body weight for a lifetime. Other diseases impact the healthy heart, however, such as heartworm disease, dental disease and certain viruses and bacteria. Regular vaccines, heartworm testing and checkups are intended to promote your dog's health and prevent many potential problems. If your veterinarian discovers an irregular heartbeat or murmur, periodic visits, an electrocardiogram and a cardiac ultrasound may be advised. Just as in human medicine, cardiac medications and surgery are available to treat your dog.

Heart failure can occur in dogs with previously diagnosed heart problems, but it can also happen to dogs that were not considered at risk. Signs of possible heart failure can be confused with other diseases, such as respiratory infection, but may be suspected if the following are present—

- shortness of breath—rapid and shallow respiration,
- coughing—particularly in the evening and overnight,
- pale pink or bluish tongue—associated with shock or oxygen depletion,
- exercise intolerance—decrease in stamina, coughing, wheezing, easy exhaustion, bluish tongue, fainting, loss of consciousness,
- unusual heartbeat—rapid and weak, rapid and pounding or unusually slow.

If your dog has developed any of the signs described above, call your veterinarian to have your dog seen within twenty-four hours. If your dog is extremely lethargic, unable to rise and generally weak, see a veterinarian *immediately*. It is of vital importance to keep a dog in heart failure as calm as possible. Speak softly, drive carefully and do not panic. If your dog is unconscious, with or without a history of heart disease, check for heartbeat and breathing:

With regular exercise and a controlled diet, dogs can maintain a healthy body weight, which contributes to a healthy heart.

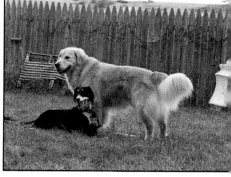

1. If heartbeat and/or respiration is absent, administer cardiac massage and/or artificial respiration as necessary—continue CPR en route to the clinic *immediately*.

2. If heartbeat and respiration are present, continue to monitor during transport. Cover your dog with a blanket and transport *immediately*.

Exposure and Other Environmental Injuries

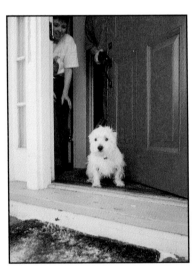

Your dog is exposed to many hazards when outside. Temperature extremes, for example, can be more than uncomfortable for your dog. He can suffer from serious heatstroke and hypothermia if left out in bad weather. Other dangers can be avoided by keeping your dog on a leash unless within a very secure area.

Attack by Aggressive Wildlife

Contact with wildlife can harm your dog in a number of ways.

RABIES

One of the most serious effects of being bitten by a wild animal is the possibility of contracting rabies. Rabies is a virus that is transmitted by direct contact with the secretions (primarily saliva and blood) of infected animals. Rabid animals do not necessarily fit the image of the frenzied and agitated beast that froths at the mouth; the infected carrier may be only subtly affected at the time it comes in

contact with your dog. This disease is fatal and it is also highly contagious to people. Speak with your veterinarian and find out what your dog requires in the way of rabies vaccines and the interval between vaccinations. Keep these vaccines updated according to the recommendations in your area. Note that rabies is currently reported everywhere in the United States, but there are regions where it has

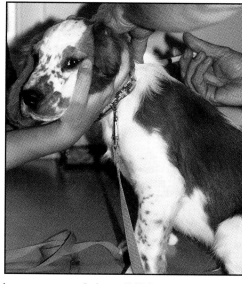

Rabies is a fatal disease. Keep your dog's vaccines up-to-date.

reached epidemic proportions—some of the wildlife that may harbor this virus include the raccoon, fox, skunk and bat, but you should know that all mammals are vulnerable to rabies, from chipmunks to moose.

WILDLIFE WOUNDS

Even if your dog survives the attack and the animal is not rabid, bite wounds and scratches must be treated as if the offending wildlife was infected with the deadly rabies virus because the risk is too great to do otherwise; also, these wounds have a high rate of bacterial infection and could require prolonged and painful treatment. Another virus that is transmitted by raccoon bites can result in a temporary but no less serious or frightening condition that may paralyze your dog—call your veterinarian if your dog comes in contact with a raccoon. If your dog is attacked by a wild animal, use gloves and act quickly to disinfect any visible wounds with warm water and plenty of soap. Regardless of whether you detect an open wound, contact your veterinarian as quarantine and a rabies vaccine booster may be required. Please refer to other relevant topics elsewhere in this book, such as "Lacerations" (chapter 3), "Disinfecting Wounds" (chapter 2) and "Applying Bandages and Splints" (chapter 2).

Drowning

Although most dogs will instinctively do the "dog paddle" in water, dogs can and do drown. Some dog breeds, like many of the retrievers, were bred to be strong swimmers. However, even the strongest swimmer may fade in high seas, panic after falling through thin ice into a frozen pond or be swept away in the current of a flooded river. A dog can drown in just a few inches of water because he need only aspirate enough water to obstruct the passage of air to the lungs. A dog could drown in his own backyard if left unattended in the swimming pool. Note that a sedated dog is particularly at risk for drowning, and a dog that is immersed to control heatstroke may survive his hyperthermia but not its treatment without careful handling in the water used to cool down his body temperature.

Even a strong swimmer may fade in high seas.

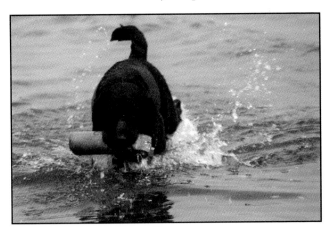

FALL THROUGH ICE

If your dog has fallen into a frozen pond or lake, call for local authorities to help with his rescue. Tie yourself to a nearby tree or have someone hold you and stretch your body flat against the ice; reach for your dog with your hand or use a rope or leash that you can loop around his neck to pull him from the water.

FALL INTO OCEAN

If your dog has fallen into the sea, use a pole to hook onto him. With a life preserver or life vest secured to the boat with a rope, you may decide to jump into the water to rescue your dog. Make certain that your own safety is secured before jeopardizing your own life in order to save your dog. When reaching to pull your dog from the water, circumstances may prevent you from grasping the back of his neck; grab onto any part of the dog that you can and do not let go—you may not have another chance.

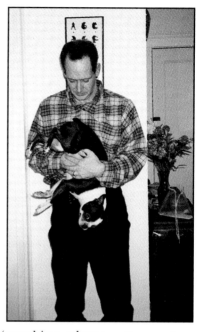

BACK ON LAND

If your rescued dog is conscious, towel him dry and keep him warm;
watch for any difficulty breathing (coughing, wheezing) or any decrease in appetite or level of activity. Near-drowning complications include polluted water and debris in the lungs, and contact with bacterial or toxic contaminants. Any problem in the several days after a near-drowning experience should be reported to your veterinarian.

If your small- or medium-sized dog is not breathing, lift him upside down and compress his chest with a quick squeeze to expel water and debris.

If your dog is unconscious when he emerges from the water:

1. Check his heartbeat and respiration; if both are present, towel him dry, cover him with a dry blanket and transport him to the nearest veterinary facility *immediately.*

2. If heartbeat is present but the dog is not breathing: Lift a small- or medium-sized dog upside down and press his body flat against yours, wrap your

arms around his chest and squeeze firmly and quickly release. Alternately, hold the dog upside down firmly by the hips and swing him in a wide arc from side to side. Repeat either process several times to expel water and debris that may have entered the airways; lay the dog back down on his side and pull his tongue forward to check his mouth for any material in the back of his throat. If the dog is too heavy or awkward for you to lift, lay him on his side with his head hanging downward; place both hands on the dog's chest with open palms and depress firmly downward and quickly release. Repeat several times as described above, removing any fluid or debris that may have collected in the dog's throat.

Check again for both heartbeat and respiration; proceed with artificial respiration with or without cardiac massage (see chapter 2).

Lay a large dog on his side with his head lowered. Compress the chest with a quick squeeze and then release.

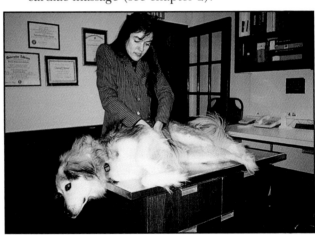

3. If heartbeat and breathing are absent, begin CPR. If the chest does not rise and fall with each assisted respiration, repeat your attempts to clear the airways with external pressure—continue CPR and transport to the veterinary hospital *immediately*.

Electric Shock

Electrocution can occur inside as well as outside your home. Live wires can fall within reach of your pet and lightning can strike dogs, too! Mischievous young dogs commonly chew on wires and cables as they explore their environment or when there is nothing more attractive on which to gnaw.

Injuries from contact with electricity include burns (blackened skin, raw sores) at the lips, tongue and gums; burns at the point of contact (feet, back, nose, almost anywhere); infection; cardiac arrhythmia/arrest; respiratory arrest and fluid in the lungs.

If your dog has received an electric shock it is essential to give priority to life-threatening injuries. Do not worry about a burn, no matter how severe, if your dog's heart has stopped. You must act cautiously but quickly.

1. Evaluate the situation: Is your dog still in contact with live electric current? *Do not touch your dog until he is removed from the source of electricity!* If your dog is unconscious or awake but unable to move, use a non-metal object (such as a broom handle or a toilet plunger) to push your dog away from the source. If your dog is conscious and able to walk, call him to come to you and away from the source of electricity. Turn off power to the offending electric source before entering the area to rescue or treat your injured dog and call the power company or fire department for help.

2. Check for heartbeat and respiration and administer CPR as necessary. Call for immediate assistance

AVOID ELECTRICAL INJURIES BY PET-PROOFING

With young dogs in particular, an important part of pet-proofing your home is to eliminate the risk of electrocution. Look around each room and think of ways to decrease the desire and opportunity to reach electric cords or wires:

- Cable covers may be purchased at hardware stores, computer stores or through specialty catalogs.

- Rearrange furniture to create obstacles to wiring, electric plugs and wall sockets.

- Place baby guards in unused wall sockets.

- If necessary, prevent access to rooms that seem hazardous with baby gates or keep the door closed.

- Place upside-down mouse traps that will snap shut to startle the curious pup and create a negative association with the electric cords near attractive wires.

- Give your dog rawhide bones of appropriate size on which to chew and make sure that he has enough daily exercise and playtime to become tired and content.

Addressing
Emergencies

and transport your dog to the animal hospital *immediately.*

3. If your dog seems uninjured but is unusually quiet, call the clinic to let them know you are on the way; dangerous cardiac arrhythmia (irregular heartbeat) may be undetectable to you and must be corrected *immediately.*

4. If your dog seems to be active and alert but has sustained minor burns to his body surface, refer to chapter 3 for the discussion of treating burns. Carefully monitor your dog over the next several hours and maintain watchfulness for several days in case complications should develop. Any change in your dog's behavior or appearance warrants a call to your veterinary clinic for further instructions.

Dogs are less likely to chew on electrical cords if they have an appropriate chew toy.

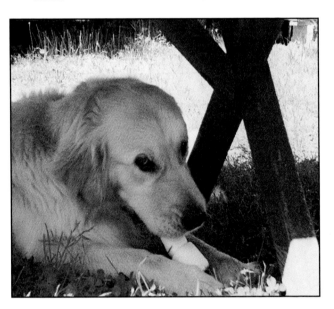

Ingestion of Foreign Object

Young dogs are notoriously curious and investigate the world around them by tasting, gnawing and playing with objects in their mouth—sometimes swallowing inappropriate objects. Some mature dogs will do the same.

If you witness the ingestion of an inedible object, there are three options:

1. Do nothing: An object smaller than ½ inch in diameter and with a smooth surface may pass through uneventfully. There are, however, unsafe items that fit this description. Coins, particularly pennies, can corrode in the acid environment of the di-

*Keep your trash
baskets inaccessible.*

gestive system and release toxic metals. Tablets or pills prescribed for your own use could be toxic to your dog; induce vomiting (see below) and call your animal hospital for further instructions, or call the National Animal Poison Control Center at 1 (800) 548-2428.

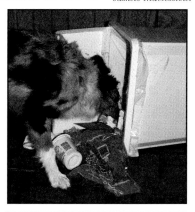

2. Induce vomiting within fifteen minutes by sprinkling a teaspoon of salt or hydrogen peroxide on the back of the dog's tongue. Do not induce vomiting of pointed or jagged items that could cause serious injury on the way back up.

3. Call the animal hospital and tell them you are on the way with your naughty pup. Depending on what the object is, how long ago it was swallowed and what the radiograph or ultrasound shows, your veterinarian may induce vomiting, use special equipment to extract the object under anesthesia or perform emergency exploratory surgery.

Repeated vomiting may be caused by swallowing a foreign object, but may also be caused by a variety

PUT SMALL ITEMS OUT OF YOUR DOG'S REACH

The importance of pet-proofing can not be over-stressed.

To prevent your dog from swallowing inappropriate objects, place them out of his reach or store them away until the dog is more trustworthy and mature. Be particularly vigilant about small items such as decorative items, children's toys and sewing kits. Remove objects that are attractive to chew such as pens, pencils, gloves, shoes, hairbrushes and remote control devices, among many more. Empty trash baskets daily or, better yet, keep them inaccessible by whatever means are necessary to protect your dog.

of other maladies (see the discussion of vomiting in chapter 6).

Hit by Car

If your dog has been hit by a car, give priority to the injury that would be fatal if left unattended. For example, a scraped elbow or broken tooth is less important than a fractured pelvis, which is less urgent than cardiac arrest; arterial bleeding from a lacerated ear is less crucial than hemorrhage from a major vein in the leg. Always eliminate the possibility of an injury that is truly life-threatening by first evaluating the vital signs:

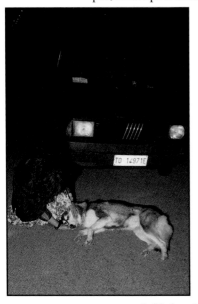

If your dog has been hit by a car, first evaluate his vital signs.

1. Check for pulse and respiration; administer CPR as necessary.

2. Control bleeding with direct manual pressure until other materials become available (ice, tourniquet, veterinary care).

3. Keep the dog covered with a blanket or towel unless he is agitated. If the dog is conscious, reassure him with a calm voice and soothing tone. You can react emotionally later, once your dog is delivered to the clinic for evaluation and treatment.

   Note: Details on administering CPR, controlling bleeding and treating a dog for shock are set forth in chapter 2.

4. Even if your dog seems fine, proceed directly to the veterinary hospital; remember, many injuries may be silent and could be delayed.

Heatstroke

Heatstroke is an abnormally high body temperature (over 104°F) caused by prolonged exposure to a hot environment. A dog that is left out in the sun on a hot summer day without access to shade or water, or forced to exercise beyond his natural capacity in the heat is at risk of heatstroke. It is also a common event in dogs that are confined in a car in direct sunlight. Never leave your dog unattended in a parked car, even if the windows are rolled down a bit. He will be safer and more comfortable at home. In any situation where there is inadequate ventilation and overheating, heatstroke may result in a real life or death emergency.

Signs of heatstroke include a body temperature higher than 104°F; fatigue, disorientation, lethargy and collapse (which may progress to seizure); vomiting and diarrhea; hyperventilation and heavy panting and very red gums (blood vessels will be very dilated at the surface to help give off more body heat). If your dog is showing most of these symptoms and has been in a situation that put him at high risk for heatstroke, you must act quickly to reduce body temperature:

1. Measure his rectal temperature and verify it every fifteen to twenty minutes during treatment to monitor his progress.

2. Place him in the bathtub in enough water to cover his body or put him in the shower and turn on cool water. Support his head above the water in your hands (in advanced stages of collapse the dog may be too weak or unconscious and could drown).

TO PREVENT HEATSTROKE

Do not insist on running with your dog or taking him on very long hikes in hot weather. Exercise should be moderate.

If you have a brachycephalic breed (flat-nosed face) such as a Bulldog, Pug or Pekingese, be extra-considerate. These dogs do not tolerate heat well.

If you must travel with your dog, make frequent rest stops for water and carry drinking water for your dog. Offer him a drink frequently.

Give your dog an ice cube as a treat!

Do not leave your dog outside without shade and clean, cool water; never leave your dog outside and unattended for longer than a half hour and check on his whereabouts every few minutes.

Provide an inflatable children's wading pool for your dog; many dogs love to lie in these on a hot day!

Let your dog run through the water sprinkler when you water your lawn, or keep him cool with a brief shower from your garden hose.

3. Alternatively, aim the garden hose directly on the dog, being careful not to aim the spray at the dog's nose or mouth.

4. Place ice packs at the pads of the feet in order to cool the dog down quickly.

5. Drape an ice pack or bag of frozen vegetables on the dog's head for a few minutes at a time until his rectal temperature reads normal.

Too much time in the sun on a hot day can lead to heatstroke.

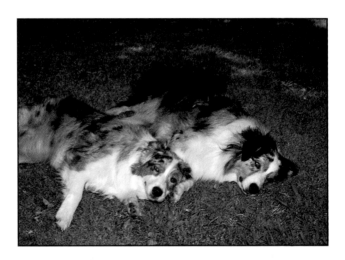

Note: If the dog is not vomiting and is alert, you may offer him an ice cube to eat every few minutes; do not offer water to the dog until he is able to move with relative ease. When the dog is ready to drink, give him ¼ cup of water every fifteen minutes to be sure that he does not drink excessively and vomit.

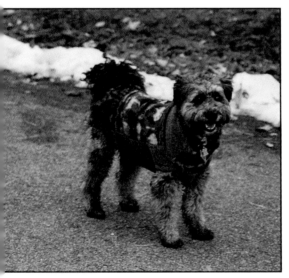

Dogs can enjoy cold weather when properly attired!

If your dog's temperature drops to normal range (below 103°F) and he seems to have fully recovered, call the animal hospital to report the incident and ask for further instructions. A professional evaluation may be called for, depending on the circumstances that created the heatstroke and the general health of your dog.

Despite your intervention, if your dog's temperature fails to decline at all within the first twenty minutes, if he has lost consciousness and does not respond in this time frame or if convulsions and tremors occur, take him to the nearest clinic *immediately*.

Hypothermia

Hypothermia is an abnormally low body temperature. A body temperature lower than 99°F is hypothermic and the dog should receive emergency care. If the core temperature falls below 95°F the dog is unlikely to recover. Prolonged exposure to cold and freezing temperatures, shock and excessively long periods immersed in water cooler than normal body temperature can cause hypothermia.

Shivering and trembling are the body's way of generating additional heat. In severe hypothermia, the dog may no longer be able to defend against drastic reduction in body heat, particularly if he is in the deep stages of shock. If your dog has been lost, missing or exposed to cold weather and seems extremely fatigued, cold to the touch, has pale gums or any sign of shock (see chapter 2), you should:

1. Cover him with a towel that has been warmed in the dryer, an electric blanket (medium heat) or a thick blanket. Gently rub his legs and body to stimulate circulation (unless other injuries make this impractical).

2. Measure his rectal temperature (described in chapter 2).

3. Surround his back and belly with several plastic containers filled with hot water or hot water

> ### HOW TO PREVENT HYPOTHERMIA
>
> Don't leave your dog in a parked car when temperatures fall. Temperatures under 50°F may be very hard on a dog, especially if he is very young or getting on in years (the exception may be the Nordic breeds—such as Huskies, Samoyeds and Alaskan Malamutes, but even these dogs have their limits to tolerating harsh climates). Do not leave your dog outdoors for longer than a half hour, even in your backyard, when temperatures dip below freezing. Some dog owners have confidence in heated dog houses, but most dogs would prefer to stay indoors with you and your family where they belong and deserve to be. Do not hesitate to "dress" your shivering dog for the weather so he can be more comfortable outdoors; many dog breeds have short coats (and several have no hair at all!) and are bred for milder climates but still need daily exercise and fresh air.

bottles (avoid heating pads unless covered with a thick towel or unless used for brief periods, because incapacitated animals cannot move away if it is too hot and could be burned). If necessary, cover your dog's body with your own—if the dog is small enough (and does not have any injury that precludes this) you may wrap him inside your own clothing to better share your body heat.

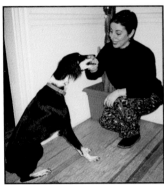

An ice cube is a nice treat, especially on a hot day!

4. Measure rectal temperature every fifteen to twenty minutes; the dog's body temperature should reach the low normal range (about 100°F) within the hour. If it does not improve substantially, if the dog remains immobile and does not shiver or if there are any other injuries apparent or suspected, see a veterinarian immediately.

chapter 6

Head and Brain Problems

Clearly, injuries to your dog's head and neurological events require a quick response. Do not hesitate to take your dog to an emergency clinic under these circumstances.

Ear Emergencies

Trauma, foreign objects and infection are the most likely causes of urgent ear problems. Trauma can lead to lacerations (cuts) or puncture wounds, which are discussed in detail in chapter 2). Even with minor wounds, injured ears frequently bleed quite a bit, partly because the dog tends to shake her head and disturb clot formation!

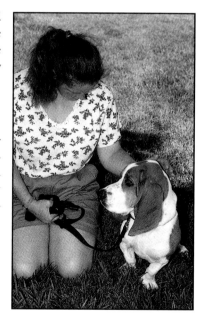

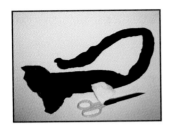

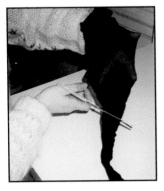

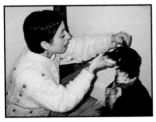

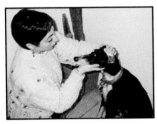

Make an ear bandage with panty hose. Slide it over your dog's face until it fits around her head, securing the injured ear and gauze dressing close to the head.

TRAUMA TO THE EAR

In addition to cuts, ear infections, insect bites and skin parasites can lead to traumatic injury of the ear. By repeated head shaking or scratching, blood vessels can be broken in the pinna, or ear flap, and cause a pocket of blood between the skin and the ear cartilage referred to as an aural hematoma. These tubular swellings on the ear flap, secondary to trauma or infection, are not dangerous to the dog but may require nonemergency surgical repair. The aural hematoma will heal without surgery, but the ear may be rippled and twisted in appearance (the equivalent of the "cauliflower ear" of professional prizefighters). The underlying infection must still be seen by a veterinarian as soon as possible.

If your dog's ear has a bleeding injury:

1. If the wound is minor and bleeds slightly, disinfect the wound and apply direct manual pressure. Apply topical antibiotic; if any signs of infection develop or if bleeding cannot be controlled, see your veterinarian the same day.

2. If the wound is large or bleeding is not easily controlled, apply an ice pack along with direct manual pressure. Next, apply several layers of gauze squares to the injured site and fold the ear flat against the top of the dog's head. Make a bandage with an old sock (cut off the toe seam) or a length of lady's panty hose and slide it over your dog's muzzle and face until it fits around the dog's head, holding the injured ear in place. Pass two fingers under the sock/stocking bandage to make sure it is not too

tight. You can remove the bandage if it seems to make your dog anxious. Call the clinic for an appointment the same day.

If your dog develops a swelling on her ear flap:

1. Apply an ice pack to the ear for at least fifteen minutes several times a day until she can be evaluated by a veterinarian; call the veterinary clinic for the earliest possible appointment.

2. Examine the inside of the ear and look for any kind of discharge, redness, odor or discomfort when you touch the ear.

3. Look inside the ear canal for any small object or debris (leaves or soil, for example) that may have fallen inside—flush with warm water as discussed below.

4. Examine the outside of the ear for the presence of insect bites along the ear margins; ticks adhered to the skin anywhere near the ear, head or neck and fleas or signs of fleas in the region of the head or neck. Treat with appropriate medication from the animal clinic.

If your dog's ear swells, look inside the ear canal for a small object or debris.

If your dog's ear seems to be very itchy, give a single dose of Diphenhydramine, an over-the-counter antihistamine, to provide immediate relief. This works particularly well for insect bites and may help temporarily for minor infections as well.

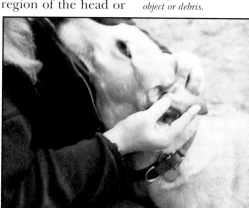

Seek veterinary attention if any ear problem persists for more than twenty-four hours.

EAR INFECTIONS

If your dog suddenly begins to scratch her ear, shake her head or rub her ear against the ground, it is possible that a foreign object has fallen into the ear canal. Lift the ear and examine the ear canal, using a small flashlight from your first aid kit. Remove any small object that may have fallen inside. If you cannot see anything or cannot reach what you find, flush the ear canal with several tablespoons of warm water—if something floats closer to the surface, use a tweezers to gently extract it (the eardrum is angled deep within the canal and you will not perforate it!). If you are unable to extract the foreign body, call the clinic to be seen the same day.

Ear infections can develop quickly or gradually but, either way, can become an emergency if the dog is extremely uncomfortable. If your pet is continually shaking her head, scratching at her ears, crying, has a fever, stops eating, loses her balance, seems unsteady and/or is walking in circles, make sure that she is seen within twenty-four hours. If your dog seems to have a minor ear infection, with symptoms such as redness, swelling, discharge, odor or pain in her ear(s), call for the next available appointment (within forty-eight hours).

Eye Emergencies

Dogs' eyes are sensitive, and those with prominent eyes are especially at risk of injury.

The dog's eye is a sensitive and beautiful instrument and is one of the most delicate organs in the body. Nonspecific signs of ocular pain or discomfort include blinking, squinting, refusal to open the eye, increased

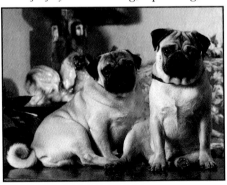

tear production and unusual discharge. The normal defense of the eye is to protect itself with the blink reflex and defenses becomes exaggerated when the eye is damaged. *Any persistent eye problem, regardless of how minor it may seem, you should receive veterinary attention within twenty-four hours.*

The major causes of ocular emergencies are trauma, foreign bodies, autoimmune problems and infection. These may involve the eyeball, the eyelids, the conjunctiva (the inside lining of the eyelids), the cornea (the clear surface layer of the eyeball) and the retina (the back of the eye). Any of these structures may be lacerated (torn), ruptured, punctured and may also hemorrhage. The eye socket may be fractured. The "white" of the eye (sclera) can become bloodshot, hemorrhagic or bumpy. Bacterial infection can invade a traumatic injury or complicate a viral infection.

Glaucoma, one of the leading causes of blindness in dogs, can occur spontaneously, but it can also follow ocular infection or traumatic injury. In glaucoma, the pupil (the adjustable opening that focuses light onto the retina) can become fixed in extreme dilation and the eye becomes painful, bloodshot and bulges as the internal pressure of the eye rises to produce a true ocular emergency.

OCULAR DISCHARGE

A dog's eyes produce clear tears that normally stain a deep mahogany color when they dry. Abnormal eye discharge ranges in color from white (usually mucus) to shades of yellow or green:

> ### KEEP YOUR DOG'S HAIR OUT OF HER EYES
>
> By trimming the hair around your dog's eyes or combing it off the face, you may decrease the incidence of irritation and possible infection. In any event, doing so will certainly enable you to monitor the condition of the eyes so that any developing problem can receive rapid attention. Preventing emergencies can be as important as, or more important than, knowing how to respond to one. Examination of a dog's injured eye can be challenging and if your dog becomes aggressive, do not insist on examining it further. Instead, call your veterinarian and have your dog seen the same day.

1. If the discharge is accompanied by fever, sneezing, coughing, loss of appetite, lethargy, itching or pain, the dog should be seen within twenty-four hours.

2. An ocular discharge with little or no sign of discomfort may be treated by flushing the eye once every six to eight hours in a twenty-four hour period with 2 or 3 drops of saline solution or sterile water. If there is little or no improvement after this time, however, contact your veterinarian without delay.

3. If the surface of the eye appears inflamed (bloodshot) and the inflammation persists for more than twenty-four hours despite flushes with saline, call

for an appointment within twenty-four hours. If the inflammation is accompanied by discomfort of any kind, have the dog seen sooner.

FOREIGN BODY

If your dog suddenly seems to be blinking rapidly, squeezing her eye shut and the eye is tearing heavily, she may have a foreign body in her eye. Even small things, such as a speck of dust or an eyelash, can cause considerable inflammation.

1. Gently separate the eyelids and examine the eyeball surface. Look inside the lining of the eyelids for any conspicuous material (you may see a filament of thick mucus that has formed around a small foreign object to protect the eye).

2. Instill several drops of saline eyewash to flush the eye; alternatively, a bottle of your own contact lens solution or clear, cool water from the tap is appropriate. Use a cotton ball soaked in water and squeeze it over the eye surface.

3. Separate the eyelids as best as you can. If you see the irritating material and it does not flush out, gently pry it out with a wet cotton ball. If your dog struggles and becomes increasingly agitated or irritated with you, leave her care to the professionals and have your dog seen right away.

4. If the eye seems less irritated after thorough flushing and the dog is comfortable, it is reasonable to wait an additional twenty-four hours before visiting the veterinarian. However, if minor discomfort persists, the dog should be seen as soon as possible. Clearly, if the discomfort is significant, either to you or to your dog, she should be taken to the clinic right away.

Note: Do not attempt to remove a foreign body that has penetrated the eye (not just floating on the surface); take your pet directly to the veterinarian. Do not risk causing additional damage or pain if foreign material is not easily extracted!

Cuts

If there is a laceration to the eyelid, flush away debris with clear water (taking care not to flush debris into the eye itself). Apply ice directly to the cut eyelid, even if there is little or no blood, to minimize swelling (the eye and associated structures swell easily and the swelling alone increases discomfort and may prevent thorough examination). Call the clinic and tell them that you are on your way with a traumatic eye injury.

Cornea Problems

The cornea (the invisible, clear "skin" of the eyeball) may suffer from lacerations, punctures, foreign bodies, autoimmune diseases and infections. Suspected corneal problems should be evaluated within twenty-four hours. Symptoms to watch for include:

- Blinking, squinting, refusal to open the eye;
- increased tear production, unusual discharge;
- white or gray spots, patches or streaks on the surface of the eyeball;
- blood vessels that seem to creep over the surface of the eyeball or superficial changes in pigment (corneal invasion by pigment cells turns it brownish-black—these inflammatory changes develop slowly over many days and weeks).

Eye Loss

Among the most shocking of emergencies is the eyeball that has been forced out of the eye socket (proptosis). This occurs most typically from blunt trauma. Proptosis can be partial or complete:

1. Do not try to replace the eyeball yourself!
2. Cover the eyeball and exposed eye socket with a sterile square gauze bandage that has been soaked in saline or water, preferably at room temperature.
3. Keep your dog calm and proceed directly to the nearest veterinary clinic.

Regardless of how ghastly a traumatic eye injury may appear, it is important to note that the same hazardous situation that injured the eye may have caused other injuries that are far more ominous. The eye is not a vital organ if the dog is in cardiac arrest or is bleeding heavily from a laceration in her leg. As discussed elsewhere in this book, always evaluate the possibility of an injury that is more life-threatening. Priority must be given to the injury that would be fatal if left unattended.

MAKE IT A HABIT TO EXAMINE YOUR DOG'S MOUTH

Routine examination of your pet's mouth at least once each month is a good habit to acquire. You need not forcefully pry her jaws apart. Lift the lips or hold on to a favorite chew toy while your dog gnaws at it. Look for firm and uniformly textured gums, clean teeth and normal pigment and breath. If there are any sudden or progressive changes, you will be able to recognize them. Watch for unusual positions of the tongue or jaw, constant licking movements, foul mouth odor, thick and constant drooling, bleeding, pawing or rubbing at the mouth or muzzle, gagging, coughing, pacing, restlessness and refusal to eat or drink. Call your veterinarian for the earliest available appointment today. If your dog is showing any of these signs and becomes aggressive when you try to examine her mouth, do not insist any further—leave it to the professionals!

Oral Emergencies
BLEEDING FROM THE MOUTH

Bleeding from the mouth may be caused by trauma or a foreign body, but can also be due to the loss of "baby teeth" (deciduous or "milk" teeth) in pups or dental disease in adults. Pups lose their "baby teeth" between 4 and 6 months of age and, although they are usually swallowed with little bleeding, the canines and molars can sometimes bleed a bit. Bleeding due to tooth loss is no cause for alarm in pups but should receive attention in dogs over 6 months old that have their adult dentition. A fractured tooth is open to infection and jagged edges may harm the dog's mouth. If your dog's teeth appear encrusted in plaque, stained, cracked, broken and bloody or her gums seem to be unusually swollen, tender and bleed easily, schedule an appointment for a checkup as soon as possible. If these symptoms are accompanied by a fever or a decreased appetite, have your pet seen within twenty-four hours.

Gum Pigment Changes

Many dogs have mixed gum pigmentation and may normally have pink, pinkish-brown and black areas. Changes in pigment, from pink to black or from black to pink or white, should be brought to your veterinarian's attention. Malignancy in the mouth may be more typically tumor-like but can also be a subtle change in pigment. Schedule a checkup at your earliest convenience.

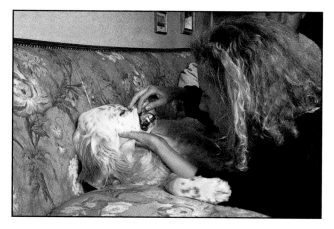

Make it a habit to examine your dog's teeth and mouth including gum pigment changes.

Choking

Choking occurs with complete obstruction of the back of the throat (pharynx) or upper airways. This might happen if a ball, mouthful of food or a thick plug of mucus or saliva is inadvertently aspirated.

A choking animal cannot vocalize or make any sound at all. It cannot whimper, whine, growl or bark because no air can pass from the lungs outward across the vocal cords to produce sound. A choking dog will make gagging movements with neck outstretched, mouth open and the tongue becoming increasingly blue. Extreme distress will be followed by collapse and unconsciousness within minutes. Respiratory arrest is the direct consequence of airway obstruction. Without immediate intervention, cardiac arrest follows.

Artificial respiration (and, therefore, CPR) will fail in a choking victim unless the obstruction is removed. It is critical to remove the obstruction to restore the airway. There are four basic techniques to dislodge obstructed foreign bodies in a dog's mouth or throat:

1. Check the inside of the mouth and throat. This step is reserved for the unconscious dog that is not breathing and for when the chest does not inflate during artificial respiration. If the dog is still conscious, proceed to the alternative techniques that follow. Do not stick your hands into a choking dog's mouth when she is in a state of panic. You risk unnecessary injury to yourself and will only exacerbate the dog's condition. As difficult as it may be, wait until the dog loses consciousness to explore her oral cavity:

   • Pull the tongue forward and downward toward the dog's chest to dislodge any item that may be there.

   • Reach with a bent index finger into the back of the dog's throat to feel for any object or material that might be obstructing the airway.

   • If you see an object but cannot reach it, use a spoon or tweezers to do so, but be careful not to push it farther into the airway.

   • Be prepared to administer CPR immediately following removal of the obstruction.

2. The Heimlich maneuver is appropriate for conscious and unconscious choking dogs:

   • Stand behind the dog and encircle her chest with your arms.

   • Lift the dog's torso so that her back is against you.

   • Make a fist with one hand so that the knuckle of the thumb rests against the dog's body and cover it with your other hand; position your cupped hands in the middle of the belly just below the rib cage.

   • With a sharp, upward thrust, squeeze your cupped hands into the dog's belly and release.

- Repeat if necessary; the obstructed object should be expelled with force.

- Check for heartbeat and breathing; administer CPR as needed and get veterinary help immediately.

3. An alternative method is to lay the conscious or unconscious dog on her side:

  - Place the palm of one hand on the chest over the last few ribs and cover it with the other hand.

  - With a sharp, downward thrust, press into the dog's chest and release.

  - If the dog is unconscious and the object is not visibly expelled from the mouth, open the mouth and sweep the back of the mouth and throat with a bent index finger in case the obstruction has dislodged but remains in the oral cavity.

  - Check for heartbeat and breathing; administer CPR as needed and get veterinary help immediately.

4. A final method is simply to hold the dog upside down with her belly facing away from you. Encircle her hips with your arms and swing the dog back and forth—this is most effective when combined with the methods above, alternating as necessary to restore a patent airway.

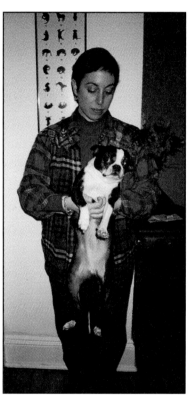

To perform the Heimlich maneuver, position your hands (hand over fist with thumb pressing inward) in the middle of the belly just below the rib cage.

Note: The following variation of the Heimlich maneuver applies to unconscious choking victims *only* and may be attempted if other methods fail: Hold the dog upside down and drape her body over the back of a straight-backed chair so that her head hangs

109

downward. Position her belly just below the rib cage over the top of the chair back; lean your body into the dog's legs to pin her between you and the chair, or pass your shoulder under the dog's hips. Reach your arms around to the dog's back and with a quick squeeze press her into the chair and release; the obstructing object should drop to the floor.

Coughing

Coughing occurs when the respiratory system is irritated (such as from smoke or chemical fumes inhalation), infected, infested (such as with parasitic worms) or inflamed (autoimmune or allergy-related responses). Coughing can also be due to a buildup of fluid in the lungs and airways that occurs when the heart fails to function normally, for example, in heartworm disease or heart failure.

Coughing is not the same as choking. Intense coughing can progress to bouts of choking, however, even when the airway is not obstructed. Coughing is a symptom of a problem and is only urgent if the cause of coughing is harmful. If the coughing is due to an upper respiratory infection, for example, it is not an emergency. If the coughing is due to smoke inhalation because the dog was rescued from a burning building, it deserves immediate attention.

If your dog's cough began within the last week or so and she was recently kenneled, groomed professionally or hospitalized at a veterinary clinic for another matter, she may have an upper respiratory infection (a "common cold" to us). The best places to catch the viruses or bacteria that cause "a cold," are those where other dogs are frequently found and where the dogs remain in close contact with each other.

If your dog's cough is accompanied by sneezing and/or teary eyes, she probably has an upper respiratory infection that could be contagious to other dogs. Keep her confined to your home and yard; make sure that her vaccines are kept current every year through her lifetime.

If your dog is coughing but seems otherwise unaffected (alert, good appetite, active and playful as usual), wait a few days to see if the coughing improves; if coughing persists or worsens, call for a checkup without further delay.

If your dog is coughing and has a fever, decreased or no appetite, seems sluggish and withdrawn, anxious or uncomfortable, call for an appointment within twenty-four hours.

If your dog coughs mostly or exclusively in the evening or overnight, cardiac disease should be considered among the list of possible causes. Call for an appointment as soon as possible (sooner if your dog's health or attitude seems affected in any other way); speak with your veterinarian about recommendations for heartworm detection and prevention in your area.

Convulsions

A convulsion, also referred to as a seizure or "fit," is a sudden and involuntary muscular contraction or series of muscular contractions. A convulsion may last for a few seconds or it may continue for many minutes. It may affect only a small body area (petit mal seizure or Jacksonian seizure). For example, the dog may appear to stumble or her jaw may chatter uncontrollably for a brief moment. If a seizure is caused by abnormal electrical activity in the emotional centers of the brain (such as during a psychomotor seizure), a sudden mood swing of aggressiveness may be triggered. Convulsions can also cause the dog to collapse and lose consciousness during massive and violent spasms. Occasionally, major generalized seizure activity will continue for prolonged periods (grand mal seizure) and require intensive veterinary care.

A seizure may happen just once or only a few times and never recur. Alternately, seizure activity can occur sporadically over a lifetime or convulsions can progress and become more frequent, more intense and longer in duration. If seizures are a symptom of a disease, it is important to try to identify the cause of the seizure in case the illness can be treated. If seizures are due to epilepsy (abnormal zones of electrical activity in the brain) or to untreatable causes, anticonvulsant (anti-epileptic) drugs may be recommended for the remainder of your dog's lifetime.

If your dog is already on anticonvulsant medication and has a seizure that is worse than usual or has a cluster of seizures within a single day or several days, call your veterinarian for advice or have your dog seen right away (depending on the severity of the episodes). The goal of these medications is to reduce the number and severity of seizures. To cure seizure activity completely is the ideal outcome but is usually not realistic, especially in primary epilepsy.

If you think that your dog is having a seizure, *do not put your fingers or anything else in her mouth!* Your dog will not "swallow her tongue" during a convulsion but you could be seriously injured by the involuntary movements of her jaw.

1. Move the dog only if she has collapsed in a precarious place, such as at the foot of the stairs, near a swimming pool or in the street.

2. Do not cover her with a blanket—body temperature rises during convulsions and excess body heat should be allowed to escape.

3. Look at your watch and try to time how long the seizure lasts. This could be helpful information for your veterinarian.

4. After convulsing has stopped, verify heartbeat and respiration. If heartbeat and/or respiration are absent, administer CPR and seek veterinary attention *immediately*.

5. If the dog's heartbeat and respiration are stable, measure her body temperature. If her rectal temperature is elevated (up to 104°F is not uncommon immediately after a seizure), pour cool water over the pads of your dog's feet every few minutes and recheck rectal temperature after fifteen and thirty minutes to make sure that she has begun

to cool down (stop when her temperature is under 103°F).

EMERGENCY CONVULSIONS

Your dog should be brought to see a veterinarian *right away* if:

- your dog has collapsed into generalized spasms that continue for longer than five minutes;

- her tongue takes on a bluish hue during or after the seizure;

- she has any difficulty breathing during or after the seizure;

- she does not rise long after muscular contractions have disappeared (in the few moments after convulsions have ceased, your dog may remain dazed for about fifteen or twenty minutes and may seem tired for a few hours afterwards) or continues to be unusually lethargic longer than three hours after the seizure;

- rectal temperature is over 104°F one hour after the episode is over and your dog is still very lethargic;

- she has a second seizure within twenty-four hours;

- she has been previously diagnosed with any of the illnesses known to cause convulsions listed above.

Coma

Coma is complete loss of consciousness. The dog may appear to be asleep but *cannot be aroused.*

If you discover that your dog is unconscious and cannot be revived by calling her name or rubbing your knuckles on her rib cage:

1. Verify the presence of a heartbeat and respiration; administer CPR if needed.

2. Determine whether your dog has suffered a head or spinal injury. If this is suspected, transport with great care, using a stretcher if possible.

3. Control any obvious bleeding injury.

4. Go to your veterinarian's office *immediately.*

Fainting

Fainting (syncope) occurs when consciousness is suddenly and momentarily lost. Your dog may faint if the brain's oxygen supply drops, for example, when the heart rhythm is abnormal and blood is not pumped efficiently. Fainting itself is not a real emergency; however, the reason underlying the episode may become one. Did the dog simply stumble and fall, or did she have a brief seizure or some other neurological or cardiovascular condition? Perhaps the dog merely lost her balance because of an inner ear problem. If heart failure is responsible for the loss of consciousness, then the dog eventually could develop urgent symptoms associated with cardiac disease. Fainting also can become an emergency if the animal injures herself while falling, perhaps because she fell in an awkward position or tumbled down the stairs. Head injuries and lacerations, for example, may be consequences of fainting.

Unlike these sleeping puppies, comatose dogs cannot be revived!

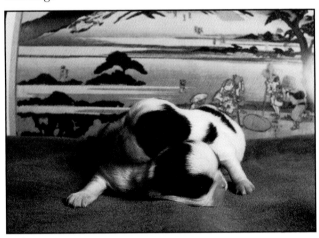

If your dog suddenly drops down to lie on her side or her belly: Call her name to see if she responds to you. Are the eyes open or closed? If the eyes are open, does she blink when you pass your hands before her eyes?

If the dog is simply dazed, reassure her with your voice to keep her calm and give her a few moments to recover. If the dog seems all right, schedule a checkup as soon as possible.

If the dog does not respond to you, rub her rib cage with your knuckles briskly to stimulate a response; if the dog regains consciousness but is unable to rise within five or ten minutes, have her examined by a veterinarian right away.

If the dog does not regain consciousness when you rub her rib cage, *immediately* check for heartbeat and respiration; administer CPR if necessary, cover with a blanket and transport her to the veterinarian's office *immediately*.

Bone
Injuries

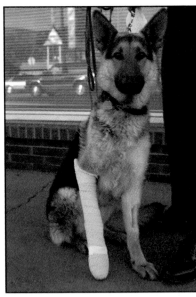

Bone injuries can be very serious and are always painful. If you think (or know) that your dog has suffered a broken bone, try to remain calm and remember to approach your dog with caution.

Broken Bones

There are two major categories of broken bones, or fractures. An open fracture is one in which the bone fragments protrude at the skin surface.

A closed fracture remains hidden beneath the skin but should be suspected if an animal is unable or reluctant to bear weight on the injured limb. A fractured tail may hang limply or be pressed tightly between the legs.

Closed fractures can be extremely damaging. A fractured rib, for example, could puncture a lung, or lacerate the heart. A fractured skull can be fatal.

Closed fractures are further classified as "stable" or "unstable." In a stable fracture, the bone fragments remain relatively interlocked and normally aligned. If the fracture involves a limb, the dog may even attempt to walk. This type of fracture must be distinguished from severe sprains, dislocations and other soft tissue inflammation that can be, at least initially, as disabling as a broken bone. In general, however, the pain of broken bones will deter voluntary movement of the limb. A stable fracture may not be visible on radiographs (x-rays) until several days after injury. A fracture is unstable when the bone fragments are out of normal alignment and function is impossible.

FIRST AID FOR AN OPEN FRACTURE

If your dog has an open fracture or wound:

1. Pour sterile water *only* (no antiseptic of any kind) over the surface to flush away dirt and debris. Avoid touching the wound with anything but the water and the dressing that will follow. Be careful not to dislodge bone fragments that might be viable for fracture repair and do not touch the bone or wound with your hands.

2. Apply a nonstick sterile dressing, if possible, and cover with a light bandage.

3. If the wound is bleeding, disinfection is of secondary importance. An ice pack can be placed over the sterile dressing and loosely bandaged around the site. If bleeding is profuse, you may need to apply a tourniquet.

4. Place a folded towel beneath the limb during transport. A lightweight splint (such as cardboard or newspaper) may be helpful for added stability during transport as well as to prevent further damage and pain; however, a splint is not essential.

5. See a veterinarian *immediately*. (See chapter 2 on how to transport a pet that cannot walk.)

First Aid for a Closed Fracture

If there is a closed fracture:

1. Apply ice (optional) and a splint (limbs only); alternatively, loosely apply a very thick bandage (not tight, just thick—the layers will provide support and prevent swelling) to provide cushioning during immediate transport.

For some injuries, such as an open fracture, the best splint may simply be a folded towel placed under the limb during transport.

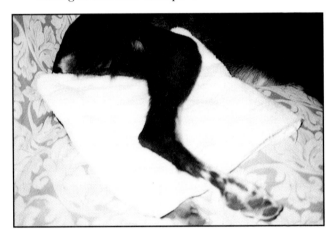

2. If your dog resents manipulation of the injury, *leave it alone.* Place a folded towel beneath the limb during transport.

3. See your veterinarian right away. There may be nothing you can do other than to transport your dog to the nearest veterinary facility, especially if your dog has broken his jaw, skull or spine.

Limping

Limping, or lameness, implies an uneven gait. Laceration, infection, foreign body, joint disease and tumors are some of the problems that may affect the canine leg from toenail to shoulder blade. Limping also may be caused by congenital problems such as chronically dislocating knee caps (chronic patellar subluxation). In addition, neurological disorders and autoimmune disease may produce limping. Limping may appear gradually and remain unchanged or worsen progressively over many days and weeks. The latter condition would be typical of arthritis or a growth that impedes movement. Limping can also appear suddenly (due to a stone embedded between the toes or a sprain, for example) and be associated with varying degrees of discomfort or pain.

Lameness is considered mild if the dog still bears weight on the affected leg most of the time but normal motion is impeded. Moderate lameness is associated with intermittent nonweight-bearing positions such as frequent stops to sit and rest, or brief pauses to raise the

> ### DO NOT TRY TO RESET A BONE
>
> Regardless of the type of break your dog incurs (open or closed), do not try to reset a broken bone yourself! You could cause additional damage and complicate the injury!

leg off the ground. A limp is severe if the dog is unable or unwilling to bear weight on the leg. Some dogs may be very stoic when in pain and will not utter the slightest whimper until you touch the spot that hurts. Be careful when you examine an injured leg in case you unintentionally harm your dog and he instinctively tries to defend himself. At the other extreme, some dogs will scream in apparent agony for relatively minor problems. It is important to keep your wits about you and remain as objective as you possibly can when your dog is in trouble.

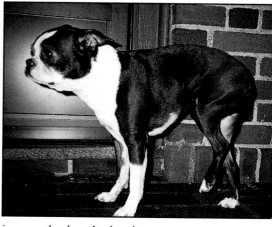

Although there are many reasons why a dog might become lame, the same basic approach applies to most cases. Evaluate the whole dog first before focusing on the leg. Is the dog alert, breathing well and behaving normally? Attend to the most serious condition first. If your dog's leg was injured because he was hit by a car, for instance, it is far more important to look for signs of shock or to address profuse bleeding than to examine the injured leg. If your dog is fine except for lameness, you may proceed to examine his leg more closely.

Moderate lameness is associated with intermittent nonweight-bearing positions.

119

First Aid for Lameness

Systematically check the affected leg from the bottom to the top of the limb.

1. Closely examine the dog's feet:

   - Hold the paw, without squeezing or twisting it, and gently separate the toes to examine between them; do the same under the foot and examine each foot pad. Look for any crack or cut on the foot pads or the skin between them.

   - Make sure there is no red, moist or swollen area, or any unusual odor.

   - Check for the presence of any penetrating splinter or foreign object, such as a sticky burr or insect stinger.

   - Examine the toes one by one for broken, bleeding or infected toenails. (See the discussion in chapter 5 concerning paw injuries.)

2. If you find no obvious reason for lameness (and even if you do), wrap your hand around the dog's leg. With gentle pressure moving upward toward the shoulder, feel for any swelling, painful area or wound between the foot and the shoulder. Apply first aid as needed.

3. Sudden lameness associated with moderate or extreme discomfort, loss of appetite, laceration, puncture wound, swelling (with or without discharge), suspected fracture or fever should be seen by a veterinarian on an emergency basis. Apply first aid appropriate to the situation (e.g., ice pack for swelling, direct manual pressure for bleeding or a splint for a fractured limb).

4. If your dog is limping just a bit but seems otherwise unaffected (he has no visible wound, normal temperature, appetite and behavior), it seems reasonable to wait two or three days before a veterinary examination, to see whether the problem resolves on its own. During that time, however, you should:

- Restrict your dog's exercise (walks on leash and for short distances) for at least three days.

- If the lameness persists beyond just a few days, seems to be getting worse or is affecting your dog in any other way, call to schedule a veterinary appointment within twenty-four hours.

Lameness frequently signals pain in dogs and should not be allowed to continue when timely diagnosis and appropriate treatment could relieve the discomfort. Any persistent, continual or intermittent change in gait, regardless of your dog's age, should be brought to your veterinarian's attention. Call your veterinary clinic to report your concern about any problem, no matter how minor it may seem, for additional recommendations.

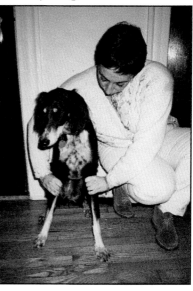

Spinal Injuries

The spine is a column of many small bones called vertebrae that are loosely fitted together. It begins at the base of the skull and extends to the tip of the tail. The spine functions to encase the spinal cord. Between each vertebra are the intervertebral disks, which act as cushions to buffer the vertebra during movement and to protect the delicate spinal cord.

Systematically check the affected leg—compare the legs to detect any changes on the injured limb.

Spinal problems that may result in emergency situations include infections, trauma and congenital diseases that may affect the vertebrae, spinal cord or intervertebral disks. These may result in intense pain or no pain, spastic motion or paralysis, chronic degeneration or even instant fatality.

Infections of the spinal cord and column are most commonly due to viruses and bacteria, although other infectious agents may be the cause. These infections may be diffuse over the length of the spine, such as in

121

meningitis, or they may be local, such as abscesses. The dog may or may not develop a fever but he is almost always in considerable pain. Depending on the nervous pathways that are impacted, the dog's ability to move or to feel may be affected.

Traumatic injury to the spine can result in dislocation or fracture of the vertebra or disks. This in turn may cause hemorrhage and swelling of the spinal cord and nerve branches and result in temporary or permanent nerve damage. Trauma may also sever the spinal cord. A severed spinal cord at the neck is often fatal. A severed spinal cord below the neck may result in paralysis. Traumatic injury to the tail is often painful but will have the least significant consequences. Traumatic spinal injuries in dogs are most often related to being hit by motor vehicles, but can

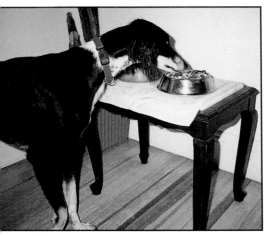

Dogs with a history of neck injury should eat and drink from elevated surfaces to promote healing.

also occur by falling from heights or in dog fights. Overzealous use of choke collars can also injure a dog's neck. These should not be used on small dogs or dogs with slender necks. Used correctly, choke collars are meant to deliver a quick "jerk and release," but no more than that.

Spinal injuries may be indicated if your dog holds his neck rigidly and slightly downward and resents moving quickly. He may refuse to eat or drink altogether, or he may eat or drink only if the bowls are elevated off the floor. Your dog may refuse to jump onto or off the bed or sofa as usual, hesitate to walk up or down stairs or cry when he jumps in or out of the car. Another sign of a possible spinal problem is the development of progressive incontinence (especially fecal incontinence in aging German Shepherd Dogs).

Also look for whether your dog has difficulty walking in a straight line or seems to stumble, wobble or swagger (especially at the hind legs), whether he is very slow to rise or to lay down again, whether he holds his tail down persistently or resents having his tail lifted. Finally, note whether your dog reacts in pain if his head, neck or back is touched.

If your dog shares any of these symptoms, call your veterinary clinic for an appointment today. Your veterinarian will need to exclude the possibility of many other conditions with the same or similar signs. If your dog has been in any type of traumatic situation, bring him to a veterinary facility *immediately.*

FIRST AID FOR A DOG UNABLE TO RISE

If your dog is unable to rise and remains lying down:

1. Evaluate the dog for the presence of heartbeat, respiration or a hemorrhaging wound—administer CPR or apply a pressure bandage as necessary.

2. Cover him with a blanket if he is unconscious or shows any signs of shock.

3. Lift your dog slowly and carefully (one arm under the shoulder and head, the other just in front of the hip bone to keep the spinal column as immobile as possible).

4. If possible, slide a stretcher or blanket under your dog for *immediate* transfer to the clinic. If you do not have a stretcher, do not remove your dog from your vehicle when you arrive at the clinic—notify the staff of your arrival and they will take care of the rest.

part three

Beyond the Basics

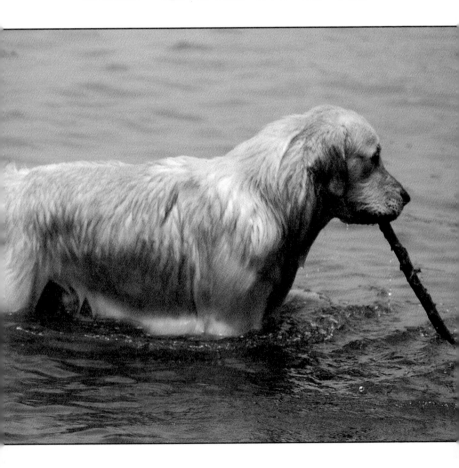

chapter 8

Recommended
Reading

About Health Care

Bamberger, Michelle, DVM. *Help! The Quick Guide to First Aid for Your Dog.* New York: Howell Book House, 1995.

Carlson, Delbert G. and James M. Giffin. *The Dog Owner's Home Veterinary Handbook.* New York: Howell Book House, 1992.

Evans, Mark. *Dog Doctor: A Guide to Common Ailments and Treatments.* New York: Howell Book House, 1996.

McGinnis, T. *The Well Dog Book.* New York: Random House, 1991.

Schwartz, Stefanie. *Instructions for Veterinary Clients: Canine and Feline Behavior Problems* (2nd ed.). New York: Mosby-Year Book, Inc., 1997.

Schwartz, Stefanie. *No More Myths: Real Facts to Answer Common Misbeliefs about Pet Problems.* New York: Howell Book House, 1996.

UC Davis School of Veterinary Medicine Book of Dogs: A Complete Medical Reference Guide for Dogs and Puppies. New York: Harper Collins, 1995.

About Training

Ammen, Amy. *Dog Training: An Owner's Guide to a Happy Healthy Pet.* New York: Howell Book House, 1995.

Ammen, Amy. *Training in No Time.* New York: Howell Book House, 1995.

Baer, Ted. *Communicating With Your Dog.* Hauppage, NY: Barron's Educational Series, Inc., 1989.

Benjamin, Carol Lea. *Dog Problems.* New York: Howell Book House, 1989.

Benjamin, Carol Lea. *Dog Training for Kids.* New York: Howell Book House, 1988.

Benjamin, Carol Lea. *Mother Knows Best.* New York: Howell Book House, 1985.

Benjamin, Carol Lea. *Surviving Your Dog's Adolescence.* New York: Howell Book House, 1993.

Dibra, Bashkim. *Dog Training by Bash.* New York: Dell, 1992.

Donaldson, Jean. *The Culture Clash.* Oakland, CA: James and Kenneth Publishers, 1997.

Dunbar, Ian, PhD, MRCVS. *Dr. Dunbar's Good Little Dog Book.* James and Kenneth Publishers, 2140 Shattuck Ave. #2406, Berkeley, CA 94704. (510) 658-8588. Order from the publisher.

Dunbar, Ian, PhD, MRCVS. *How to Teach a New Dog Old Tricks.* James and Kenneth Publishers. Order from the publisher; see address above.

Dunbar, Ian, PhD, MRCVS, and Gwen Bohnenkamp. Booklets on *Preventing Aggression; Housetraining; Chewing; Digging; Barking; Socialization; Fearfulness* and *Fighting.* James and Kenneth Publishers. Order from the publisher; see address above.

Evans, Job Michael. *People, Pooches and Problems.* New York: Howell Book House, 1991.

McMains, Joel M. *Dog Logic—Companion Obedience.* New York: Howell Book House, 1992.

Rutherford, Clarice and David H. Neil, MRCVS. *How to Raise a Puppy You Can Live With.* Loveland, CO: Alpine Publications, 1982.

Volhard, Jack and Melissa Bartlett. *What All Good Dogs Should Know: The Sensible Way to Train.* New York: Howell Book House, 1991.